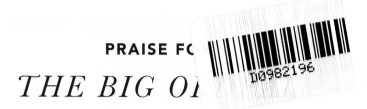
"*The Big Ordeal* addresses a critically important need for cancer centers and their patients to better understand the emotional arc of the disease and how to support patients through what is a physically and psychologically challenging experience."

—STEVEN K. LIBUTTI, MD, FACS, Director, Rutgers Cancer Institute of New Jersey; Senior Vice President, Oncology Services, RWJBarnabas Health; Vice Chancellor Cancer Program, Rutgers Biomedical and Health Sciences

"While important strides in cancer care have led to substantial increases in survival, the personal experience of having cancer remains extraordinarily challenging. In *The Big Ordeal,* Cynthia uses her knowledge as a cancer patient and her skills as an observer to present a message of understanding and hope for all those touched by the cancer experience."

—GREG FRICCHIONE, MD, Professor of Psychiatry, Harvard Medical School; Associate Chief of Psychiatry, Massachusetts General Hospital; Director, Benson-Henry Institute for Mind-Body Medicine

"*The Big Ordeal* is a vital guide for patients and family members contending with a cancer diagnosis, treatment, and life beyond. Interweaving the empathic perspectives of a survivor with grounding insights from the science of the stress response, fear, anxiety, depression, cognition, and resilience, this book provides a unique roadmap for an often disorienting and life-changing journey. With its double helix of heart and science, *The Big Ordeal* is a must-read for anyone trying to fathom the unfathomable."

—JONATHAN ALPERT, MD, PhD, Chair, Department of Psychiatry and Behavioral Sciences, Montefiore Medical Center; Professor of Psychiatry, Neuroscience, Pediatrics, Albert Einstein College of Medicine

"*The Big Ordeal* is a must-read for anyone facing cancer, as a patient or loving caregiver. Through her research with patients and experts, Cynthia brings new insights and understanding to the experience of cancer, helping to reduce the isolation, fear, and anxiety so common with a diagnosis. I witness the psychosocial challenges the diagnosis engenders on a daily basis and know that the empathy and intelligence shared in this book will help to ease the stress of a cancer care journey."

—SHALOM KALNICKI, MD, FASTRO, FACRO, Professor and Chairman, Department of Radiation Oncology, Montefiore Medical Center, Albert Einstein College of Medicine

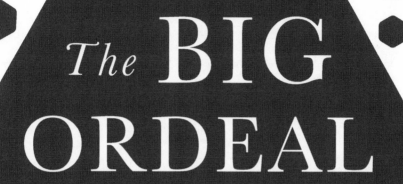

The BIG ORDEAL

UNDERSTANDING *and* MANAGING *the* PSYCHOLOGICAL TURMOIL *of* CANCER

Cynthia Hayes

Foreword and Additional Contributions by
Ann Marie Beddoe, M.D., M.P.H.,
Sara R. Pasternak, Ph.D., *and* Christian Zanartu, M.D.

RIVER GROVE
BOOKS

This book is intended as a reference volume only. It is sold with the understanding that the publisher and author are not engaged in rendering any professional services. The information given here is designed to help you make informed decisions. If you suspect that you have a problem that might require professional treatment or advice, you should seek competent help. Many of the names and identifying characteristics of the patients referenced in this book have been changed to protect their privacy.

Published by River Grove Books
Austin, TX
www.rivergrovebooks.com

Copyright ©2021 Cynthia Hayes

Distributed by River Grove Books

Design and composition by Greenleaf Book Group and Mimi Bark
Cover design by Greenleaf Book Group and Mimi Bark

Publisher's Cataloging-in-Publication data is available.

Print ISBN: 978-1-63299-335-9

eBook ISBN: 978-1-63299-336-6

First Edition

In loving memory of Amy,
with appreciation for all that she gave.

CONTENTS

FOREWORD

For twenty-five years, I was honored to take care of hundreds of women who came to a small chemotherapy suite on the Upper East Side of Manhattan for treatment of their various gynecologic cancers. As their physician, I developed a close bond with each of these women and was privy to private conversations they shared with each other as they sat for countless hours while their chemotherapy was infused.

It struck me, in listening to the women, that very little of their conversation focused on cancer. Rather, patients shared freely how they tried to cope with the lack of control, the fear, and the anxiety that a cancer diagnosis brings. They talked about how cancer was changing their home lives, their work lives, even their intimate lives. The emotional toll united these women as they recognized that they were undergoing not only a physical experience but an emotional transformation that could be felt only by those who have a diagnosis or are intimately involved with someone who does. And through their conversation, they validated one another's emotions, learned from one another strategies to deal with those emotions, and gained the strength they needed to get on with their lives.

One of these women was Cynthia. As a card-carrying member of this unique group of women, Cynthia always wanted to know the "why" and "how" of everything she experienced, physically and emotionally. As her physician, I did not have all the answers, but Cynthia was determined to find those answers, and she did—not just in her countless interviews with fellow cancer survivors, but through her in-depth research and interviews with experts in the field.

The result of her inquest is *The Big Ordeal,* which explores in detail the psychological turmoil that patients go through with cancer. It presents the typical emotional response to the disease at each phase in the process and shares the science behind those emotions and the collective wisdom of fellow patients and caregivers about managing them.

I would like to think that the chemotherapy suite was the cocoon that gave birth to this remarkable book. It provided Cynthia with an environment in which people were disarmed—they could let their hair down (or, rather, hang their wigs up) without being judged or embarrassed. It is a must-read for anyone entering the world of cancer for the first time, or the second or third time. It is a must-read for caregivers, friends, relatives, or coworkers of anyone going through the cancer journey.

—ANN MARIE BEDDOE, MD, MPH

INTRODUCTION

No one expects a cancer diagnosis. But that element of surprise, that jolt out of nowhere, becomes a defining factor in how we experience cancer, setting us up for the cascade of emotions the disease and its treatments will provoke in the weeks, months, and years to come. As unexpected as the diagnosis might be, the roller coaster of emotions that follows is actually somewhat predictable—instant panic and fear of death give way to stress, anxiety, feelings of isolation, and depression. These affect patients' quality of life, hindering their adherence to treatment and often interfering with physical recovery.[1] Angst and fear of recurrence remain constant companions for several years until either one achieves physical recovery—passing the magical five-year mark and eventually regaining emotional health—or the cancer returns, bringing with it anger, denial, guilt, demoralization, and sometimes, acceptance of the inevitable.

The Big Ordeal
The Emotional Turmoil of Cancer

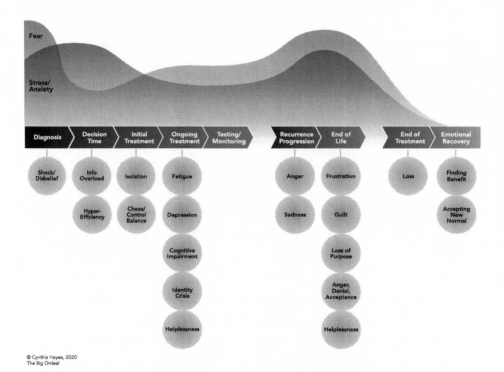

© Cynthia Hayes, 2020
The Big Ordeal

Of course, our personal histories, DNA, diseases, and treatments influence how we internalize and express our emotions, but the patterns are far more common than we might expect. Nearly 70 percent of patients report feeling stress and anxiety;[2] up to 60 percent experience fatigue, cognitive issues, or both, during and after treatment; 16 percent of patients face major depression; and 10 percent experience post-traumatic stress disorder (PTSD).[3] Although the field of psychosocial oncology began in the 1970s, it wasn't until 2007 that the Institute of Medicine (now known as the National Academy of Medicine), finally acting on what was understood about the impact of emotions on physical recovery and quality of life, established standards requiring that the psychosocial needs of the patient be integrated into routine cancer care,[4] and only in 2015 did the American College of Surgeons' Commission on Cancer mandate that screening for distress be part of a hospital's protocol in order for the hospital to be awarded accreditation.[5] Today most hospitals have some type of social-support programs for cancer patients, but emotional health is not yet a mainstream concern among oncology practitioners, particularly in the out-patient-care facilities where most patients receive treatment. In the crunch for time with their patients, and with a primary focus on eliminating the disease, medical professionals avoid emotional topics, dance gingerly around them, or stomp on patients' psyches without realizing the impact of their words. Given the cultural stigma associated with mental illness and emotional problems, we don't always feel comfortable raising the topic with our physicians or know to seek support from the social-service programs available, meaning that few of us who are newly diagnosed with cancer receive any psychological support.[6] At the same time, most books for patients avoid or only graze the surface of emotional topics, focusing instead on the physical and leaving us in the dark.

The Big Ordeal: Understanding and Managing the Psychological Turmoil of Cancer addresses emotions head-on, validating patients' feelings through survivors' shared experiences and helping patients, caregivers, and even doctors better understand the emotional ordeal, the physical and chemical drivers of those emotions, and coping strategies to get through it all.

My own ordeal started on a beautiful, blue-sky September day. My daughter and I were headed to a neighborhood salon for manicures. When my cell phone rang, I was surprised to see my gynecologist's name on the display. Having been in the week before for a regular checkup, I assumed it was someone in the office calling about a billing issue and answered as we continued walking. But I stopped short when I heard my doctor say I had flunked my Pap smear—it had detected "atypical glandular cells." Probably it was nothing, she said, but I needed to come back in for more tests. She was at the hospital in the middle of a delivery, so she signed off quickly with assurances and instructions to call the office. It went by so fast I didn't quite know what to make of her call. My daughter and I were on a mission with a deadline—we were going out in two hours and our nails were not yet red—so I carried on without giving it much thought. Moments later, sitting in the salon, I called to schedule the follow-up procedures, but the office had already closed for the day.

There are times when it might be better not to be such an insatiable internet researcher. I had just a few minutes to use my phone before succumbing to the manicurist and quickly learned that "atypical glandular cells" were the warning signs of a particular type of uterine carcinoma that had grim survival statistics. I went from unconcerned to terrorized in an instant. Cancer already had a grip on my emotions, and it would be a long weekend of grappling with the possibility that I had a life-threatening disease.

"Everything is going to be fine," my husband assured me, feeding me the same line I had taught him to say years before when he had tried to solve a problem that needed only solace. But this problem needed more than a comforting arm around the shoulder. What if I did have cancer? At fifty-seven years old, I was too young to think about sickness and death, but it seemed unlikely that the Pap smear was a false positive. I wanted to talk to someone who would understand my fears, but my best friend, the one who would have known exactly what to say to acknowledge the intensity of my feelings and be with me in the moment of foreboding, had passed away only nine months earlier from the very disease that threatened me now. I felt isolated and alone.

The endometrial biopsy the following week was excruciating, but not as bad as the wait for results. It was a week of suppressed terror—putting up a brave front and a false smile while inwardly on the verge of tears or frozen with panic. I was home alone when my doctor called with the news. "I am very sorry to tell you this, Cynthia," she said, "but the biopsy results confirm that you have cancer." The news hit with the force of a tornado, depriving me of air and upending my life. Instantly, my head ached, and my heart raced. I had cancer. And not just any old cancer, but uterine papillary serous carcinoma, an aggressive, fast-growing cancer. The nightmare I had kept under wraps for two weeks was real.

I was in shock but needed to act quickly. I needed scans. I needed to find a surgeon and schedule pre-op testing. Most of all, I needed my husband, who at that moment had a mouth full of cotton in the dentist's chair. It all happened so fast, I barely had a chance to think, let alone cry. Phone calls and emails, recommendations and confirmations. By the end of the day, I was scheduled for a morning with the radiology team for scans of my entire torso and had appointments with two surgeon candidates. The scans would give us further insight into the depth and breadth of my cancer, but not until a surgeon had probed my inner organs and removed many of them would we know the stage of my disease, a prognosis, and a treatment plan—more waiting and uncertainty, and more dread.

In the United States alone, nearly 600,000 people a year die from cancer.[7] For centuries, the disease has been synonymous with death. A diagnosis was accompanied by a timeline, usually short, and encouragement to get one's affairs in order. But improvements in screening and detection mean that many cancers are being caught in earlier stages, when they are more treatable. At the same time, breakthroughs in treatments are helping patients live longer with the disease and return to health.

But that death sentence is still what we hear when we learn we have cancer. Like the roar of an approaching train, overpowering the words of the speaker beside us, the diagnosis instantly overwhelms, blocking out information and insights that might help us understand how to deal with the disease and move forward with our lives.

I was lucky, destined to join the ranks of the survivors. Although uterine papillary serous carcinoma historically carries a survival rate of less than 40 percent,[8] my cancer was caught early. After surgery and another anxious week waiting for the pathology report, I received the good news from my doctor that it was stage 1, consisting of a small, single tumor confined to the uterus and barely dug in, which significantly increased my odds. It helped, too, that I was in New York with a top-notch care team, expert in my type of cancer. Also, I was healthy going into the ordeal and had a loving support network, all of which eased the process. Surgery and six chemo treatments later, I was cancer-free. Five years after the diagnosis, the terror is as faded as my surgical scar.

But the process from diagnosis to recovery was far from smooth and easy. While my doctors were clear about the physical effects of surgery and treatment, we had few conversations about the emotional toll the process would take. And although my family was prepared to support me through the helplessness of surgical recovery, the nausea of chemotherapy, and the cancer-induced malaise, none of us anticipated the emotional swings, the anxiety, or the cognitive impairment that accompanied the physical trials. When I dissolved into tears at my fate on the fourth day after every chemo treatment, we didn't know that withdrawal from the steroids pumped into me as part of the treatment could lead to an emotional crash, and that the despair I felt so acutely one day would be gone the next. I was told to anticipate the loss of my hair as chemo progressed but wasn't prepared for the loss of my identity as I shifted from high-functioning executive to obvious "cancer patient," with bald eyes and a blank stare—no longer on top of my game physically, mentally, or emotionally.

While I often felt adrift in my emotional turmoil, as the months passed, I was surprised to learn that I was not alone. Conversations with friends and colleagues—even with acquaintances at the gym as I struggled to regain some strength—revealed that many cancer patients experienced the same emotional volatility, the same anxiety around test time, the same relief mixed with fear when cleared, and the same urge to make something good of it when cancer was finally history. And the more I spoke with patients and survivors, the more clearly I saw the patterns in how we respond to the ordeal.

How to Read This Book

This book was written to help you learn from the wisdom of those who have gone before you, fellow travelers on a journey none of us wishes to take. Based on interviews with over one hundred patients, including those newly diagnosed, in treatment, recovering, or facing their final days, it presents real-life situations and real emotions, as well as advice from real cancer patients: things they wish they had known going into the disease, and lessons they learned the hard way.

Each chapter covers a particular phase in the process, from diagnosis through treatment and progression, recurrence, and recovery. I use patients' stories to present the most common experiences while highlighting the myriad ways of dealing with complex emotions at a time of stress. With the help of medical experts, I have written an explanation of the science behind the emotions—what's going on in your body as a result of the disease and its treatment that is contributing to how you feel—and addressed some of the related issues that arise, such as dealing with intimacy as treatment progresses, communicating with your medical team, and the emotional benefits of exercise, stress reduction, and complementary therapies.

This book is meant to be a guide. It's full of examples, information, and advice that will help you understand your psychological response and see that while you are unique, you are not alone. Feel free to underline and highlight as you go. Take note of the parts that resonate with you and come back and read them again another day. Our emotions are fluid, and what feels right one day may leave you scratching your head the next; an idea that seems ridiculous on first reading may be the solution you need when you view it again.

I suggest you take each chapter when it is relevant and don't read too far ahead. It can be overwhelming to look at the whole sequence, but by focusing on one step at a time, we usually find the strength to deal with what's before us. I also recommend that you share the book with your loved ones and those in your support network. It will help them understand what you're going through and how to help, ensuring that you get the support you need.

Whether you are newly diagnosed or struggling with a recurrence, I hope *The Big Ordeal* will give you possibilities and options that help you with your own ordeal.

SHOCK AND DISMAY: WHEN BAD NEWS HITS

"Nothing in life is to be feared, it is only to be understood. Now is the time to understand more, so that we may fear less."

—*Marie Curie*

For centuries, a cancer diagnosis was synonymous with a death sentence. As early as 3000 BCE, experts declared "There is no treatment,"[1] and patients were told to prepare for an untimely, sometimes painful death. That was still true for 50 percent of cancer patients as recently as 1975.[2] But much has changed in the intervening decades about our ability to find and treat cancer. Earlier detection and a richer understanding of the disease itself have led to significant improvements in our prospects. According to the National Cancer Institute, mortality rates from the disease fell 29 percent between 1991 and 2017 in the United States,[3] and today, five-year survival rates for the two most common cancer sites, prostate and breast, are upward of 90 percent. For the five most common types of cancer combined—which account for more than half of all new cancers—66 percent of patients now survive.[4] Even those statistics are based on history, not current or future cancers, so they underestimate our chances of recovery. Given recent advances in immunotherapy and precision medicine, which are dramatically changing how some cancers are treated, there is ever more hope for survival. Of course, no two cancer patients are alike. Health at the time of diagnosis, care teams, responses to treatment, and a million other variables differ, but a cancer diagnosis is no longer an automatic death sentence.

Despite these improvements, our gut reactions haven't changed. When we hear we have cancer, we still fear we will die. Whether it is rational or irrational, that fear is visceral, instant, overwhelming, and almost universal. Patients who are otherwise healthy and have an excellent likelihood of beating the disease burst into tears and find it hard to imagine overcoming their emotions, let alone the disease. Or they sit in stunned silence, unable to hear the doctor's reassurance or advice.

A Pocket Full of Death

Smart, outgoing, athletic, and good-looking, Carl knew he was one of the lucky ones. He had a great life. Opportunities came his way unbidden. He had a wonderful wife, Rebecca, and two young sons who were happy and healthy. They had the good fortune, the love, and the fortitude to enjoy life. "It was as if there was a protective shield around us, guarding us and keeping us safe," he said. He knew others who struggled with life or suddenly had their lives upended or run aground, but that seemed far from his reality. His was a privileged view: that life had a way of working out fine. Until he got the news that shattered his protective shield.

> Rebecca had noticed a spot on my arm that didn't match the rest of my freckles. I spend a lot of time outdoors, and given how fair I am, in my adult years I used plenty of sunscreen and had the idea that was good enough. When I went to get it checked out, the dermatologist said she thought "it was nothing," but biopsied it anyway "just to be sure," and made an appointment to share the results. I assumed that she was right. It was just a funny brown spot.
>
> When I was back in her office the following week, she said, "It's melanoma." I really must have known what melanoma was, but at that moment, I truly couldn't place the word, so I asked her, and she said just two words, "It's cancer." This was at a major academic medical center, and I wanted to know how they were going to fix it, so I asked her about the treatment. "Well, for melanoma," she said, "we have no effective treatment." She seemed uncomfortable giving me the news, handed me a referral to the local cancer center, and left the room. This was 2002, and even early experimental treatments were unproven. Right away, I assumed I was going to die. From the moment I heard I had cancer, my new reality seemed discontinuous, severed from all my life before. But at the same time, weirdly, it

also seemed like I now knew my life story, complete with ending. The idea that I had cancer and there was nothing to be done (I always knew how to take action) just flipped me out.

Carl panicked. The thought that his life was over was horrifying enough, but the idea that he would leave his wife and kids, still so young and dependent, was heart-wrenching. He tried to reach Rebecca at home and at work with no luck—she was running around making last-minute preparations for their son's middle school graduation party taking place later that evening, and no one carried cell phones in those days. Leaving the dermatologist's office, he went straight to the office of a doctor friend, hoping for some uplifting advice, but he wasn't given much solace there either. "The die is cast," he was told, leaving him even more despondent and terrified.

I walked into the party a couple of hours later and was struck by an incredible sense of isolation. Here I was in this beautiful place with the afternoon light bouncing off the river in the background, and all these happy people, so many friends, going about life as if everything was fine. No one knew what I was facing; no one could see that my whole world had changed—or what was left of it. I didn't even know if I would see my second son reach this milestone. I felt like the walking dead.

He wasn't really alone; his wife was loving, full of advice and support, his sons a constant source of energy and joy. But he felt that no one fully understood his fear, the impending sense of doom. It didn't help that he was living temporarily in Boston, away from most of his friends in his hometown, New York, or that he had left his academic job just weeks before. The lack of a daily routine created a sense of suspended animation—unstructured days spent largely alone. He used this time to research doctors, eventually finding a surgeon who gave him confidence, and a clinical trial for a new treatment, interferon. But when he sought advice about whether or not to participate in the trial, the best the surgeon could say was, "There are probably twenty experts in the world, and they don't know what to do. So you just need to do what feels right," confirming for Carl the sense that his cancer was his responsibility alone.

> I remember going down to New York to meet with the doctor who had come up with the treatment protocol for the clinical trial. I brought copies of all my biopsies, all my medical records, even the glass slides with tissue samples, and stuffed them into the pockets of my vest. I took the subway to the doctor's office and as I stood on the crowded train and patted my pockets to be sure everything was there, I felt like a suicide bomber—the weight of those samples and reports was so great, so secretive and explosive. Everyone else was going about their own business, living in their own worlds, and here I was with a pocket full of death. No one knew what I was going through or what might happen next.
>
> Back when I had just turned thirty, I came down with a potentially fatal heart problem overnight. That came out of the blue as well, and the doctors were worried, but it didn't threaten to invade other

organs. And I could at least partly understand the specialists' explanations. And, happily, it resolved in several weeks. But this was different. This was ambiguous. The medical science seemed like voodoo. This was cancer.

What is it that makes cancer so scary? Part of it is the stories we have all seen and read—the ancient history and the all-too-recent accounts of someone who didn't make it. But a big part of it is the uncertainty: not knowing if you are going to survive, not knowing what the course of treatment will be and how you will respond to it, and not knowing when—or if—you can ever feel safe from cancer again.

Most cancers can't be fully evaluated at the time of diagnosis. A melanoma, a lump in the breast, an irregular blood test, an abdominal mass—we are told they are cancer, but not what that really means. Some cancers grow quickly and seem to spread like wildfire; others are slow-growing and noninvasive, even chronic. Some require extensive treatment and never fully resolve, while others are dispatched with minor surgery or daily medication. This variability, and having to wait for days or even weeks knowing we have cancer but not yet knowing how bad it is, heightens the sense of uncertainty and fear. Further testing and scans help inform us how big, how deep, how widely spread the cancer may be, but often it is not until doctors have surgically removed the tumor, gotten "clean margins," checked adjacent lymph nodes, and received reports back from the pathology lab that they can begin to understand the true nature of the disease coursing through our bodies. Then and only then can they assess its severity, determine the appropriate treatment, and talk about a prognosis.

Gasping for Information

For Monica, the challenges at diagnosis time were more than just fear of the disease. She literally couldn't talk. A journalist in her fifties, she was used to asking hard questions, digging for information, and piecing together puzzles. She was also used to working long hours and not having a moment to take care of herself. At the time, she had been so busy with work that she had ignored a variety of nonspecific symptoms for months before finally seeing her doctor and getting a computerized tomography (CT) scan.

> When my primary care doctor got the report, all I was told was, "You have a significant mass in your abdomen. Get the first appointment you can with this doctor." They never used the word "cancer" but handed me the name of an oncologist. As a patient, you are left drawing your own conclusions. I understand doctors wanting to be circumspect when all the facts aren't there, but saying too little produces anxiety too.

Monica's visit to the oncologist the next day only added to her confusion. The doctor spent a long time telling her all the things it could be but didn't offer any clarity about what she suspected was going on. "I came away thinking there was a fifty-fifty chance I had cancer, and I didn't know how to deal with that." She maintained her relentless pace at the office while scheduling surgery and pre-op testing. That didn't leave a lot of time to focus on whether she did or didn't have cancer. But it was there in the back of her mind, adding to her general sense of foreboding.

A week later, I woke up from the operation, still intubated and unable to talk with that tube down my throat. I was so scared. I scribbled a note to my husband, who was sitting beside me, and he told me it was cancer—advanced, aggressive ovarian cancer. Instantly I thought, "Holy cow, I could die." Hearing that news and having that thought while being intubated was just awful—the panic and not being able to discuss it, and having to process it while dealing with the pain and the incision and the anesthesia, were just too much.

Monica knew all too well that cancer could change one's expectations of life. A friend had recently passed away from ovarian cancer, leaving behind twins who still needed mothering. But Monica had never imagined that cancer would interrupt *her* life. There was no family history of cancer; her father had lived to be ninety, and her mother was still going strong at age eighty-eight.

Mom came to visit me at the hospital, and as she was sitting beside my bed, I was thinking, "I always assumed I would live as long as her, that I would have at least another thirty-five years." But now I had cancer, and all bets were off. I was so afraid I was going to die young.

I kept thinking about all the things I wanted to do right away and regretting that I wasn't going to have more time with my husband, whom I had married just ten years earlier. He didn't want to even talk about the possibility that I might die. It's not that he was unsympathetic, but he was dealing with the same fear, so it was hard to have that conversation.

As pressing as her concern was, Monica discovered that nobody wanted to talk about these fears with her. Mostly people just ignored the question of mortality; she found that hard. There was one chaplain in the hospital who was willing to listen to her and let her cry, but ultimately, she realized "the only person who can confront your mortality is you."

Using her skills as a reporter, Monica set to work investigating, asking questions, and searching for information that would illuminate her future. She went online, read research studies, and tried to learn as much as she could about her cancer in the hopes that she could better understand the most important question—was she going to die from this? But none of her efforts proved satisfying.

> One of the tricky things for me to navigate emotionally was figuring out what numbers applied—what was the likely survival rate for my cancer. My doctor kept telling me not to look at the numbers, to pay no attention to the survival rates. "You are an N of 1," he said. "No one else has your body, your cancer, or your mindset. The numbers are meaningless." Maybe he was right, but that didn't make it any easier to deal with. You want to know what to expect, but all of a sudden, your life is in question.

Being forced to face the possibility of death is the underlying cause of so much angst in the first days or weeks after a cancer diagnosis. Long before all the tests come back and a plan is in place, we must confront the possibility that life may be cut short. Whether the odds are good or bad, or the cancer is caught early or late, it's impossible to know on which side of the divide you will fall, how you will fare with the treatment, and whether or not you will have the chance to get on with your life.

As much as we may enjoy the thrill of a movie with unexpected plot twists, that's not what most of us want in our daily lives. Human beings are creatures of habit. We tend to like routine and predictability—to know that our commute is going to take between forty-five and fifty minutes every day, to be able to plan a picnic based on the weather forecast. While a traffic jam or sudden downpour can ruin the day, when we hear news that calls into question our assumptions about the rest of our lives, we are shattered. Sure, the unexpected happens all the time—people do get hit by buses, after all—but it happens to someone else, not us.

Seeing Red

Brian was used to the unpredictable. Having grown up in Northern Ireland during "The Troubles," he'd seen his father's shop get bombed, his mother's office shot up, and people he had known killed. That was normal. That was the life he knew. Because of all that danger as he was growing up, he had been taught how to move quickly when threatened, and how to move on when the crisis had passed. So when cancer attacked him personally, he relied on his childhood training.

> Out of the blue one day, I was peeing red. That's not normal, and I was scared. I dropped everything and

went to see my doctor, who got me an appointment with a specialist for the very next day. That doctor told me it was probably nothing—at thirty-nine, I was too young for cancer—but did a test anyway. Results came back two days later but were inconclusive, so he said we should investigate further by looking inside my bladder. He scheduled me for an outpatient procedure the very next day.

When I came out of the anesthesia, he told me, "It's cancer, and I have removed the tumor." I just shut down emotionally and quickly switched into coping mode. "Okay, so what do we need to do?" I asked. I got very pragmatic. This was a fast-moving project that needed to be managed, I had experts to help me, and I would just do what they told me to do.

Shortly before his diagnosis, Brian had moved to New York to escape the emotional fallout of a long-term relationship that had just ended badly. He was still insecure in his new job and hadn't had a chance to build the deep friendships one would typically draw on for support at a time like this. There were people he could call to accompany him to an appointment or bring him home from the hospital, but no soul mates. And his family was an ocean away. He felt tremendously alone.

After growing up in a war zone, I had been shipped off to boarding school at age eleven, a harsh place with a lot of bullying and physical punishment—like something in a Victorian novel. There was no one there to help, so I got used to dealing with traumatic things on my own.

But this was coming at me so fast. First, the news that it was cancer, then they told me it was the most aggressive type and that I would need chemo. I couldn't process it all. I don't think I allowed myself to feel the trauma of it. I just stayed in the mode of managing what needed to be done. It was a form of emotional coping. I wasn't going to be victimized by cancer; I was going to attack it right back.

While our past experiences can affect the way we interpret and respond to stress, our fears about cancer also can be exacerbated or managed by how physicians share the information. Unfortunately, the task of conveying the bad news often is left to physicians we barely know, specialists we see because of a suspicious test result, who may not be able to establish rapport and communicate in a way that works for us. When a doctor says, "I wish I had better news," you are bound to feel a little more uncomfortable than if you hear, "You're going to be fine, but there is something we have to deal with."

Jackie was convinced that she had a sinus infection or tonsillitis when a soreness in the back of her throat persisted. She made multiple visits to her primary care physician and an ear, nose, and throat specialist before being told by her doctor, a man she had known for years, "This is not life-threatening. You will be fine. It will be a big inconvenience for six months, but you will be fine." She had to ask, "What will I be fine from?" before learning it was lymphoma, not tonsillitis. "I was worried they were going to send me for a tonsillectomy, so learning I had cancer this way just took all the stress away."

Pramod had thought he was anemic before the doctor broke the news to him. "He shook my hand and said

'Congratulations, you have one of the good cancers,'" Pramod remembered. "I had never heard of chronic myelogenous leukemia, but he said it was like having diabetes. So long as you take your medication every day, you'll be fine. That really took the sting out of it."

Those experiences are in sharp contrast to Michelle's. She was not yet forty when she felt a lump in her breast. Initially assured it was nothing, she kept pushing her ob-gyn, who reluctantly sent her to get a mammogram and sonogram, and eventually, a biopsy.

> I think I knew it was cancer. I think I was trying to convince myself it was nothing for a while. But when I went for the biopsy and the doctor said, "This is not good," it sort of freaked me out. I had a crazy schedule for work that week, so I just put it out of my head.
>
> I brought my husband with me for the follow-up visit, but the doctor didn't even show up! The office tracked her down and she called in, nonchalantly saying I had cancer, probably stage 3. "It's bad," she said. Even though I knew already, I burst into tears, and then was surrounded by a couple of nurses, who were shocked that I was crying. How could they expect that I wouldn't show emotion at a time like that?

SCIENCE SIDEBAR: MORE THAN JUST A RACING HEART

It's hard not to show emotion when we hear bad news. Our bodies are hardwired for fear. At the most basic level, animals—and that includes newly diagnosed cancer patients—have a preprogrammed response to threatening stimuli. And we've been conditioned to fear cancer. So hearing the words "You have cancer" initiates a fear response, stimulating a region of the brain called the amygdala to release the neurotransmitter glutamate, which in turn signals the hypothalamic-pituitary-adrenal (HPA) system—our internal stress regulator—to kick into high gear.[5]

The HPA system signals the body to produce and release steroid hormones, including the "stress hormone" cortisol, and a collection of neurotransmitters that help us mobilize to deal with the emergency. Cortisol makes the heart beat faster; heart rate and blood pressure go up, breathing becomes faster, and the ability to take in oxygen increases. At the same time, the digestive system shuts down and blood moves away from the skin—producing that familiar chill—and toward the heart and lungs to help us be hypervigilant and focused on the original fear-creating sensation. If we were standing on the African plain facing an approaching lion, that hypervigilance would help us detect the most minute movement and assess our need to fight or flee, but in these circumstances, it may not help us deal with a more complex type of stress.

The neurotransmitters, or chemical messengers, being

released include dopamine, norepinephrine, and epi-nephrine, more commonly known as adrenaline. These neurotransmitters communicate with the region of the brain that triggers emotional response, and we experience fear. They also signal the brain to release the neuropeptide S (NPS), which increases alertness and a sense of urgency, decreases our ability to sleep, and primes us for flight, should that be necessary—which actually makes it harder to get the rest we need to prepare for our impending cancer ordeal.

These neurotransmitters also suppress activity in areas at the front of the brain that usually govern the ability to manage the tasks of daily life—the higher-order thinking we all need for decision-making and negotiating the complex-ities of social interactions. When this activity is suppressed, it interferes with short-term memory and rational thought, making it difficult to concentrate and playing havoc with our normal sense of inhibition. All of this may make it easier to flee the lion but makes it harder to cope with a cancer diagnosis, often preventing us from hearing the additional information doctors and other care providers may be com-municating at the time of diagnosis such as a prognosis or the need for additional testing. At the same time, high levels of stress hormones can strengthen memory storage, creat-ing that vivid picture of the moment you heard the news, and can improve working memory and your powers of con-centration, helping you get through those endless phone calls to arrange your care.

During this time, the body is also releasing dopamine, which helps control movement and allows us to freeze so

continued

the lion will no longer think we are prey, but can also create a state of emotional numbness; more glutamate, which increases nerve activity and helps us have the energy kick we need in order to flee; and adrenaline, which will help us muster the strength and drive to get away from the impending threat, but doesn't help us sit still and listen with a rational, open mind. Depending on the strength of your reaction, you could find yourself startling easily at other noises, having nightmares or difficulty sleeping, being irritable, or even flying into rages.

Cortisol, the main driver in this chain of events, isn't released only when we have reason to be afraid; it is released every morning to help us get moving, and it is increased when we ingest caffeine or do intense physical exercise, or even if we are sleep deprived. Go into a doctor's appointment with high cortisol levels for any of those reasons, and you are apt to feel an even greater response to the new release of cortisol when you hear the word "cancer." At the same time, laugh at a couple of puppy videos or get a massage or go dancing, and your cortisol levels can plunge.

But it's not just external stimulation that influences the fear response. There are genetic factors and experiential or learned responses that influence how we respond as well. Some people are much more likely than others to be sensitive to fear-producing stimuli. Some have a more active response to their fears; others are more passive. Thirty years of yoga meditation or an abiding faith in a higher power will likely increase your ability to remain detached from the fear and prevent or minimize the normal flow of hormones and neurotransmitters, while trauma or abuse early in life will generally heighten your response. A strong sense of competence and confidence in your ability to manage life also tends to decrease the magnitude of the fear response or quickly bring it under control. But the presence of existing stress—from work, other family health concerns, financial woes—increases the overall load on your system, exacerbating the perception of acute stress and reducing your ability to bounce back from new stressors.[6] It can be difficult to predict how any of us will respond, but one study found that nearly 70 percent of cancer patients experience stress at the time of diagnosis.[7] That's part of what makes the diagnosis so challenging.

The variability in reaction also makes it difficult to explain our own responses to others. Since we each experience fear differently and react differently—based on our own genetics and life histories—it can be hard for even family and our closest friends to understand exactly what we are feeling and how best to respond. They may want to help but be unsure of what to say or do. Talking to others about what we are experiencing can help, though. Not only does it give loved ones a better idea of what we are feeling, but sharing has been shown to help us cope. In a study that looked at factors influencing the quality of life for cancer patients, intimate sharing about cancer is associated with greater comfort, reduced anxiety, and overall better family adaptation to the diagnosis.[8]

Fear turns into a related emotion: anxiety. Characterized by restlessness, irritability, difficulty sleeping, and trouble

continued

concentrating, anxiety is a generalized response to an unknown external threat or internal conflict. This transition occurs when the initial stimulus has passed, but the emotions haven't—the lion is gone, but the fear of lions persists, even when we're back in the city. We've regained our composure from the moment we first heard the news, doctors have explained the next steps and likely course of action, and family members have reassured us that everything is going to be fine, but we still worry about the unknown and unknowable after our cancer diagnoses. Progressively higher levels of corticotropin-releasing factor, another hormone released in the brain, stimulates a metamorphosis from a state of increased arousal and readiness for action into a state of expectancy and anticipatory fear.[9] We are ready for a pride of lions—or at least more bad news.

Anxiety tends to be a constant companion for cancer patients, who often deal with uncertainty for months or even years after the initial diagnosis. How bad is my cancer? How will I respond to the treatment? Will it cure my disease? Is that random twinge related to my cancer and a sign that it has metastasized? Will my cancer come back? What will I have to do next if it does? The HPA system remains overactive, and a fast heart rate, rapid, shallow breathing, and increased muscle tension can persist, creating a general sense of unease or even panic that interferes with our family lives and our ability to concentrate on our work or deal with social situations.

Researchers continue to gain insight into the biological bases for the fear reactions and understand where in the brain the reaction starts, which neural and chemical pathways the signals travel, and which systems are affected by the flux of physical sensations as we respond to stress. But they have yet to determine a way to predict how any of us will respond to the same threat—how intense the emotion will be and what it will feel like. However, knowing that our emotions are driven by physical stimuli, and that our bodies respond automatically to those stimuli, helps us understand that fear and anxiety are normal responses to a cancer diagnosis. The more we—and our loved ones—appreciate that this response is normal, the easier it is to share our fears and cope with the disease.

Twice the Trouble

Because it can be so difficult to predict how people will react to the news, telling loved ones you have cancer adds another layer of stress to the diagnosis. Whom do you tell, and when? How do you break the news? What do you do when they are far away? These decisions are complex and come at a time when many patients feel they have limited ability to handle one more burden. Sharing the news while protecting parents and children from its full emotional impact can be especially hard.

Mary R. faced this challenge when she learned that she had Hodgkin's lymphoma. Twenty-six years old and living far from home, she was making plans to go to graduate school in a few months when she started experiencing random symptoms. First, she developed a persistent cough. It wasn't bad, but after six months, she decided to see a doctor. He wasn't alarmed, so she wasn't either. Then she developed what her dermatologist decided was psoriasis. Nothing unusual. But when she started having back pain if she took even one sip of alcohol, she began to get a little concerned.

> About this time, I had decided to quit my job in preparation for some backpacking before starting graduate school. I was working out every day, getting in shape for a rigorous trip, but the cough was becoming bothersome. I went to a different doctor who thought I might have acid reflux. He ordered some tests, including one for tuberculosis. When that came back inconclusive, he ordered a chest x-ray.
>
> The technician was very casual when I arrived, but after looking at the first image, he came running out and asked if I was coughing blood. That's when I knew something was seriously wrong. My doctor ordered a CT scan and a lymph node biopsy for the next day, and said he suspected cancer. That was the scariest night, and I couldn't help but think about death. But I didn't feel I could tell my parents yet—what if it wasn't cancer? Whatever anxiety and fear and concern I was feeling, I knew my mom would feel it twice as much.

Mary R. had always been emotionally close to her family, but her parents and sisters lived on the other side of the country, so she enlisted an aunt to go with her for a CT scan. After the scan and biopsy confirmed that she had lymphoma, they called her parents together, with her aunt doing most of the talking.

My mom was crying so hard she couldn't speak. I was already thinking about what it meant for me and my body for the next year, not to mention the logistics of getting my job back and finding someplace to live and postponing grad school, but it was such a shock for my parents. I felt I had to hold back some of my emotions to make it easier for them. I worried about how honest I could be, given how emotional they both were, especially my mother. Later, when I woke up in the middle of the night in tears, I knew I couldn't call my mom; I just had to cry myself back to sleep.

Lulu had a similar experience when she was diagnosed with advanced breast cancer at age thirty-four. Born in Mexico City, she had come to the United States on a scholarship to learn English when she was fifteen and worked her way up from packing boxes on the night shift—so she could go to school during the day—to being named operations manager at a major book distributor.

When the radiologist told me it was cancer and they needed to do a biopsy to understand more about it, I just cried. From the beginning, I refused to think I would die, but those thoughts come to your head as soon as you hear something like that. I sat there praying for the strength to go through this, and for the right words. My mother and four-year-old daughter were sitting in the waiting room, and I had to go tell them. That was going to be even harder.

When I went out, my mom knew something was up—I had been gone such a long time. So I hugged her and told her I needed her to be strong, that I had cancer, but everything was going to be okay. She was devastated and crying so hard that my daughter, who didn't understand what was going on, started making funny faces and jokes to cheer her up. The worst was telling my husband later. He was overcome with tears, and that just broke my heart.

No Big Deal

Not everyone panics when hearing a cancer diagnosis. For some, it seems more like a rite of passage, or another of life's challenges that needs to be managed. Joy responded to a breast cancer diagnosis with nonchalance. "It didn't throw me," she said. "It was like having an appendectomy. I just did what the doctor told me to do, and it was done." Robin A. was so busy with her life and caring for others that she never focused on her uterine cancer diagnosis; later she had difficulty remembering that she had had it. "Now, when I am filling out one of those endless health questionnaires, I stop at the cancer line and have to think a moment," she said. "It isn't in my head that I had cancer."

Alan's coping style has always been denial, so he wasn't felled by the news. "What, me worry? When the first test results were ambiguous, I just clung to the idea that whatever it was, it was benign. Even when they were doing more and more tests, I told myself they were just being cautious. There was a moment of tears in my kitchen when I realized that pancreatic cancer was fatal, but even then, my rational mind kept saying 'Of course you are going to live; you have too much to live for.'"

For Sue, the threat of cancer had been hanging over her head since she was twenty-seven. Her mother had died of breast cancer that year, at the age of sixty. Sue had always been sure she would receive the same diagnosis, if not the same out-come—and felt it even more strongly as she approached the same age.

> I was keenly aware of the disease and my own vul-nerability. It was like the sword of Damocles, and I kept waiting for it to fall. Every time I went for a checkup, I worried this was going to be the one; this was the time they would find the cancer. And many times, they found something that needed to be explored further. They were always calling me back for more imaging, saying, "We need to watch this," and taking a biopsy. I'd had five biopsies already.

The extra attention and scans didn't show any cancer, but there was enough reason for concern, given Sue's family his-tory and repeated need for biopsies, that she started seeing an oncologist several years before her diagnosis. That doctor pre-scribed tamoxifen, which helps prevent hormone-dependent breast cancer by regulating the growth of estrogen; as one patient described it, "It eats estrogen for lunch." The daily pill was easy for Sue, but it didn't mean she could relax her vigilance. While it reduces the risk of breast cancer, tamoxifen comes with an increased risk of uterine cancer, stroke, and vision problems.

So when a routine gynecologic exam in the spring of 2005 showed a small cyst that was growing on her uterus, her doctor strongly recommended a hysterectomy, just to be safe. Sue scheduled the surgery for the end of July, thinking she would take a couple of weeks to recover and then be back at work. Boy, was she wrong.

> The surgery went badly, and four days after the operation I was back in the hospital. A round of tests revealed that my ureter had been cut during the laparoscopic hysterectomy, and I had sepsis. Now they needed to open me up for a much more extensive operation. By the end of the summer, I had had my fill of hospitals and languid days of recovery. All I wanted was to get back to normal life. But that wasn't meant to be.
>
> In early September, I felt a lump in my breast. There it was. I had never really expected I would dodge the bullet, but now? Despite the bad timing, when my oncologist finally said the words, "You have cancer," I felt a huge relief. I knew this day would come, and now, finally, we could deal with it.

ADVICE FROM THOSE WHO LEARNED IT THE HARD WAY

Shock, stress, tears, anxiety, denial, or even relief—emotions erupt at the time of diagnosis with surprising strength and complexity, reflecting who we are, how threatened we feel, and our diverse ways of coping. Regardless of how we internalize and express the emotion, though, most of us are left with a powerful recollection of the moment we understood we had cancer that suggests we experienced some degree of stress. Fueled by a cascade of hormones released in the moment of crisis (see the Science Sidebar in this chapter), we can easily recall the visceral reaction we had to the news, whether it was fifteen minutes ago or ancient history. For many, the emotions evoked in that moment dissolve and shift as we move into the next phase, but for others, the response to diagnosis sets the course for the rest of the ordeal.

As Carol said, "Each of us has to find our own best way to deal with cancer." But patients who have been there shared some common thoughts on how to get through those difficult first hours and days: "It really sucks," said Susie, "but you have to have to get beyond that." Or, as Deborah put it, "Experience what you are feeling. It is scary. Acknowledge that, and then move on." Anne agreed. "It's helpful to remember that most of us live. It isn't a death sentence, and it's not a judgment or a punishment. It's just a disease."

How do you move beyond the shock? Some take an aggressive stance, as Lulu did.

"Obviously, you are going to cry and be upset and be mad, but at some point, you need to stop, you need to concentrate your mind on getting ready to fight, with victory as your goal," she said. Others prefer a more measured approach. Mark said, "You can't swallow the whole thing in one bite. Take baby steps; worry about just one thing at a time." But no matter what, it seems to help to recognize that there will be good days and bad days ahead. As Fatima said, "It's going to be a roller coaster ride, but keep your faith up and do what you need to do." And many patients counsel, as Charlotte did, "You are stronger than you know you are. It's not easy, but it's not terrible either." Still, no one is expecting you to be stoic about it. Nancy H. said, "You don't have to be a super-woman about it. It's normal to be scared, so go with what you need, what feels right to you."

Often, what feels right is relying on others for support. "Don't be afraid to share it," said Deborah. "So many people don't want to talk about it, but when you allow people in to share it with you, it makes it less scary." Nina agreed: "Surround yourself with supportive people. You don't need people who aren't helpful. You need to stay positive and not go to the dark side."

Or, as Robin A. said, "Find some support, whether it's family, close friends, or an online support community of others who have been there. It really helps."

And with the support of others, seek out the best possible care. "Get the best medical care that you can," said Diane. "You have to do a little digging, a little homework."

Jill R. agreed. "Talk to friends and doctors and people who have been there to gather as much information as needed," she said. "Information is powerful."

"But don't scare yourself," cautioned Loretta. "Every cancer is different."

SIDEBAR: GOOD INTENTIONS, BAD RESULTS

When people hear devastating news about a loved one or a friend, they, too, can feel shocked and blindsided. They want to offer support, say something comforting, and do the right thing, but may not know what to say or how to show they care. Without thinking, they repeat statements they have heard or said before:

"Everything's going to be all right."

"You're strong. You'll get through this."

"Let's not panic until we're sure we have to."

While meant to be encouraging, comments such as these can negate the very real fear a newly diagnosed patient is feeling, landing more like slaps in the face than the show of support they were meant to be. Patients often just want someone to recognize that they are afraid—that cancer is scary, and their feelings of terror are valid.

Monica had lots of friends and family support when she got her diagnosis, but that didn't mean everything she heard was supportive. "The last thing I wanted was someone tell-ing me 'Of course you are going to get better, it's all going to be okay'—it's just so insensitive and denies the mortality issue staring me right in the face," she said. "Even the off-hand comment about the irony of me getting cancer when I was the one who always took care of myself wasn't really helpful. You have no control over who gets cancer or who is going to die from it."

Rachel recounts feeling disconnected from her husband

continued

at the time of her melanoma diagnosis. "He desperately wanted to be the one who was there for me but was missing the point all the time. I was scared, and his telling me not to worry wasn't going to make that fear go away."

Sometimes a spouse has a particularly hard time finding the right thing to say, in part because of fears about the personal implications of the diagnosis. If a man's wife is diagnosed and the center of his universe—the one most loved, the one most relied on for strength and support—is facing a life-threatening disease, and his world seems about to unravel, where can he even turn to talk about it?

"My wife saw things so differently than I did," Carl said. "She was trying so hard to make things work, but she didn't understand my fear, my depression. I became more dependent, which I hated. She also offered the latest random advice from her friends. Like, 'it's too much stress.' The illness put a lot of pressure on our relationship."

Many patients want friends and family simply to acknowledge the dreadfulness of the diagnosis. "Just say 'Cancer sucks, I'm sorry,'" said Jeremy, a forty-six-year-old First Sergeant recently retired from the US Air Force with life-threatening cancer of the appendix. "One guy said to me, 'Well, we all gotta go sometime.' It was so insensitive—as if he had already given up on my life."

Often, listening is as important as speaking. "Cancer is so huge. You can't assume anything about an individual's experience or reaction unless you ask. But you have to be prepared to listen," suggested Elyse, battling a rare type of lymphoma. "Just show up and be present. Don't try to fix things or pity them. Just be with them."

It's hard for people who haven't been through it themselves to understand the fear associated with a cancer diagnosis, which is why so many patients find solace in online or in-person peer support, both through individual mentoring and in groups. Whether broad-based or specific to a particular kind of cancer, peer support allows patients to share real and raw emotions and to find support for getting through the physical and psychological trauma of cancer.

"I joined the online support group Bladder Cancer Café," said Brian, "and stayed on for a long time after the initial stages of the disease. I found it incredibly reassuring to be in touch with others going through the same thing and felt very bonded to the people in the group; they offered support, advice, research insights. There's a lot of help out there, even if you can't find what you need from family and friends."

For those looking for support, the American Cancer Society's Cancer Survivors Network is a great place to start. And there are online support groups specific to most types of cancers. Many hospitals and cancer centers offer in-person support as well. One-on-one counseling, peer-to-peer programs, group discussions, and active therapy such as writing or exercise programs are increasingly available for cancer patients. If you or a family member needs support, ask your doctor for local suggestions, or check out the list of cancer-support networks in Resources at the end of this book.

CRUNCH TIME: MAKING DECISIONS UNDER DURESS

*In the end, the hard decisions
inescapably involve
imponderables of intuition,
prudence, and judgment.*

—John F. Kennedy

Across cultures and millennia, people have always placed themselves in the hands of healers. From shamans and apothecaries to the white-coated physician of today, we have long recognized their wisdom, accepted their expertise, and trusted them to cure us. But as Western culture evolved to question authority, and as individualism became the norm, our relationship with medicine began to change. Doctors no longer withheld diagnoses, patients started to ask about options and seek second opinions, and the concept of shared decision-making—a collaboration of medical expertise with patients' values and preferences—began to take off. In the past twenty years, the number of patients—particularly cancer patients—wishing to delegate their decisions has declined; today, the majority of us want to play an active role in our care decisions.[1] And that can be overwhelming.

While still struggling with the cascade of emotions precipitated by a diagnosis, we are faced with many decisions that need to be made in order for us to move forward with treatment. Most of us need to find new doctors, weigh options among treatment plans, and navigate complex alternatives in unfamiliar territory. Whom do I trust? Which doctor, treatment protocol, and approach do I think make sense for me? Who can help me through this ordeal? What can I say to family, friends, bosses, and others about my cancer, and from whom do I need to keep it a secret? How can I get the most from my insurance to cover what's necessary? What can I do to fulfill my work and family obligations while dealing with the disease?

Yet, at a time when we need to function with a high level of efficiency and courage, many of us are overwhelmed and in a fog. As Catherine put it when she had to make decisions about her breast cancer, "There are so many variables, and you are in a state of crisis. How can you decide?"

Following Instructions

Under the best circumstances, we are guided through the decision-making process by a trusted doctor with the appropriate expertise who takes control, makes arrangements, and prescribes a specific plan. This was certainly the case for Deborah, who had intense abdominal cramps that sent her to the gynecologist for what they both assumed was an ovarian cyst. When testing showed it was cancer, she was in shock. A divorced mother of three, sixty-three-year-old Deborah had lived alone for more than ten years and was used to managing things for herself. But this was a new level of challenge, tinged with apprehension about the seriousness of her diagnosis.

> It just floored me when my gynecologist said it was cancer. I was in la-la land and couldn't think straight. The fact that she scheduled the first appointment for me—set me up to see a specialist in Milwaukee—made it so much better. I couldn't have done it without her. Friends and colleagues made other suggestions, but the doctor she recommended was so knowledgeable and calm that I just put myself in her hands.

Alan, a sixty-five-year-old economic consultant, had a similar experience when he was diagnosed with pancreatic cancer. He had been receiving all of his medical care through one hospital system, and when his primary-care doctor called to say he'd scheduled Alan for some additional tests and to meet with a surgeon and a medical oncologist, Alan just followed his advice. "The initial meetings were so positive, I just stuck with it and never gave it another thought," he said.

But not everyone is so fortunate as to have things fall into place. Instead, we have to find our own way to the care we need, and rely on old, familiar patterns to get through this high-pressure time. Some patients, like Steve, are self-reliant, digging into scientific data and making independent decisions. "I was hardwired to be independent," he said. "Asking for help makes me feel awkward, so of course I was going to do this alone."

Others depend on family or friends. Charlotte put her trust in her daughter, knowing she would ask the right questions and come to the right conclusions. "She's in the pharma business and good at speaking with doctors, so I let her manage things," Charlotte explained. Teresa relied on friends, particularly those who had had cancer themselves. "I asked them to come with me to the big appointments and to help me think through the decisions."

Mark turned to prayer for guidance. While his sister helped him find the right specialists for his advanced liver cancer and parse their medical jargon, it was his faith that got him through. "When you have to climb up onto that cold steel operating table, you can either go it alone, or you can be there with God. I can't imagine being there alone."

Even when there's a physician offering help, the situation is not always straightforward. For instance, Cass, who got her breast cancer diagnosis two days before her sixty-first birthday, was pretty certain she didn't want to follow the advice of her gynecologist to be treated at the local community hospital. She felt he had let her down by not detecting the cancer sooner. "I had a family history of lobular cancer, and he never asked about it or gave me anything other than basic mammograms, even though that type of cancer can be hard to detect without sonograms," she said.

Instead, she took copies of her scans to two different academic medical centers, both with excellent reputations for dealing with her disease, and let time guide her choice.

> Even though lobular cancer isn't usually fast growing, I knew I wanted to get things taken care of right away. There was no point belaboring it. My attitude

was, "Okay, I've got cancer; let's fix this thing." I just
wanted to get on with life. So when one of the hospitals called with a surgery date the following week,
I just did it.

Elizabeth H. received different recommendations from her
gynecologist and from the radiologist who diagnosed her breast
cancer, both of whom she viewed as trusted advisors. Initially,
she thought it would be impossible to make a choice, but the
right choice soon became clear. "I wasn't conscious of switching
from full-on panic mode to resolution, but sitting in the doctors'
offices and having the doctors treat my cancer as such a routine
case was helpful. Ultimately, it was an emotional decision—one
of the doctors was very down-to-earth and direct, which was
calming. I knew in five minutes that she was the one for me."

Desperate to Get Started

Speedy resolution is not always an option, however. Jane M.
found this out the hard way when she had a hysterectomy for
what she and her gynecologist thought were perimenopausal
fibroids. A finance executive and an avid kayaker who spent
forty or more days a year paddling through rapids and steering
clear of the rocks, she could handle any challenge the water had
to offer. But the stress of learning she had a rare uterine cancer
called leiomyosarcoma, or LMS, made the most-difficult rapids
seem like a backyard pond by comparison.

I went in to have what I thought was a simple surgery and came out with a cancer diagnosis. The

shock of the news sort of empties your brain and robs you for some period of time of an ability to think—to process or query the way you previously would have. I don't think I would have believed that if you had told me, absent experiencing it. Just when you need them most, you lose your abilities.

The bad news sort of straggled in from there. It took more than a week for the lab to confirm what the cancer was. Then my gynecologist referred me to someone who was on vacation. Once I knew I had to do something, I wanted to get started. But because my cancer was so rare, finding the right expert and the right treatment plan took forever. That was the most stressful time.

This was not Jane's first cancer diagnosis. Several years earlier, she had had a lumpectomy for breast cancer. It was a relatively easy cancer, as cancers go, and the experience gave her a little practice for the shock of this diagnosis. It also meant she already knew an oncologist who might be able to help.

When I saw him again to talk about LMS, he said, "I don't know anything about this cancer." My heart just sank. I was desperate to get started. Thankfully, he was able to recommend someone, and forty-eight hours later, I was sitting with an expert who seemed warm and knowledgeable as he laid out a plan. But before I had a chance to start treatment, I went back to my gynecologist and he disagreed with my choice, referring me instead to a doctor at Memorial Sloan Kettering.

It took another week or so to get an appointment with her, and she was clearly very competent, but she insisted on a different approach. I didn't know which made more sense, so I thought I would get a third opinion in Boston. It turned out that each of the New York experts saw more patients with my cancer in a year than the Boston hospital did in five, so what would be the point?

Jane went back and forth between the two doctors, asking questions, collecting more information, and really struggling to decide. With every day that went by, she felt greater urgency about the need to get started, and greater uncertainty about which way to go. Was it better just to get started already, or better to find *the* one best doctor? One had many more years of experience, but the other "wrote the protocol" that was considered the standard. One doctor was involved in early research on treatment for LMS; the other had produced some of the latest studies. One had been recommended by Jane's oncologist, the other by her gynecologist.

My stress kept building during this time. I needed to decide but wasn't really in a place to evaluate their technical skills. Besides, people can be technically competent but not necessarily good doctors, or a good fit. In the end, it came down to personality. I knew that I would be more comfortable working with the first doctor—he really saw me as a person, unlike the second doctor, who lost her temper when I asked too many questions. Still, it took nearly two months to get to that decision.

SCIENCE SIDEBAR: STRESSFUL DECISION-MAKING

Even under the best circumstances, many people find it hard to make choices. Whether faced with a dizzying array of ice-cream flavors or balancing trade-offs in commute time, affordability, and neighborhood aesthetics when selecting where to live, we often feel stumped, paralyzed at the thought that we might not choose correctly and have to suffer the consequences, even if it only means walking away with a lingering taste of chocolate. Why is it that decisions are so hard to make?

Scientists talk about two different types of decision-making—habitual, in which we rely on the past, and goal-directed, in which we envision the future.[2] "Gut" decisions, the ones we make without thinking, actually are built on practiced patterns stored at a subconscious level—we know we like chocolate, so we always go for the chocolate ice cream without even considering the other flavors. But they take practice. For example, when we're driving, we don't consciously think about stepping on the gas or the brake to maintain a safe distance from the car in front of us; we just do it instinctively. But remember your first time behind the wheel? It probably took a lot more concentration to make those minute adjustments, and chances are you didn't maintain a smooth speed or constant distance from the car in front.

Unfortunately, the decisions we have to make at the time of a cancer diagnosis are not ones that we can (or want to) practice in advance. Instead, they are unfamiliar, laden with importance, and directed at a specific goal—achieving the best possible outcome. This means that in addition to incorporating learning from past experiences, they require us to focus our attention, gather information, assign personal value to potential outcomes, juggle the uncertainty of short-term costs and long-term benefits, and act. Make the right decision, and we feel good about it; make the wrong one, and we are subject to regret and more anxiety.

The actual process of deciding is an individual one, influenced by genetics, past experiences, gender, personality, practice, and even our moods. Some of us are risk-averse, while others are more willing to take a chance. Some focus more on future results, others on the present. Some always want to find the best solution to minimize the opportunity for regret; others are content with one that is "good enough." Whatever our typical pattern might be, we tend to stick with it, even in times of stress or when making complex decisions.

But it's not always so simple. The way a decision is presented can significantly influence how we think it through.[3] For example, it's bound to sound more ominous if your doctor tells you there is a 40 percent chance of side effects from treatment than if you're told most patients sail through with no side effects. Same facts, different presentation. Do you make the same decision?

How we position the decision in our own minds also weighs on the process. Each health-care decision taken on its own can feel momentous, but in the context of the larger picture, the choices can seem clearer. For example, focusing on the reward for getting through an unpleasant treatment

continued

(a significant reduction in the chance of recurrence) helps us get over any fears and concerns we have about the treatment itself (possibility of side effects) and make the decision to proceed.

At the same time, moods, unrelated to the decision at hand, can influence choices by altering the subjective value we place on different outcomes. In a good mood, we tend to weigh the potential for losses more heavily and therefore make a more conservative decision. And the same holds if we are naturally fearful or anxious. But catch us on a day when we are sad or angry, and the opposite is true, leading us to make riskier choices.[4]

Researchers are still trying to understand exactly how the brain functions in making decisions, and much of what we do know comes from studies done on animals or on people playing games in a lab under various psychological or physical stresses that bear no resemblance to real-life medical crises. But some findings are emerging that can help us understand why these decisions are so difficult—and how to make the best of the situation. For instance, researchers believe a part of the brain called the prefrontal cortex (PFC) plays a key role in decision-making.[5] The PFC is involved in so-called executive functions—things such as self-control, working memory, and cognitive flexibility. This is where we solve problems and make plans, and where we weigh the pros and cons of any goal-directed decision. However, the PFC also is tightly wired to the amygdala, which, as we saw in chapter 1, plays a key role in our emotions. The PFC is not a cold, calculating, all-knowing machine; it weaves together cognitive and emotional inputs, and is subject to hormonal variations, like any other human system.

Stress has multiple effects on these systems and there-fore on decision-making, depending on its severity, whether it is acute or chronic, and whether the type of decision to be made is a gut decision we've trained for at some level or a new, goal-directed decision. Firefighters make decisions in high-stress circumstances all the time, but they have trained for many of the expected stresses they encounter and may even thrive on them. Not so the average cancer patient encountering complex medical issues such as the choice of doctor, hospital, or treatment protocol.

The good news is that when we're under stress, the amygdala releases dehydroepiandrosterone (DHEA) and cor-tisol, natural stimulants that help focus attention and increase mental-processing speed. (That's why those firefighters can react so quickly under stress.) The more DHEA and cortisol our systems release, the greater this increase in speed.[6] We are turbocharged and intent. However, even mild stress can hinder other key decision-making functions, such as mem-ory consolidation as we take in new information ("Wait, what did the doctor just say?") and working memory as we juggle information to analyze a situation ("So, option A has these side effects and option B has fewer side effects but is risk-ier, but what did I just say about option A?")[7]. This makes it harder for us to use rational skills and encourages us to make gut decisions rather than goal-directed ones—even when we have no experience on which to base the call.

Chronic stress creates still further distortions, leading us

continued

to perceive the world as more uncertain, less predictable. This seems to overwhelm the analytical mind (PFC), and we are more likely simply to throw up our hands and say we can't decide, or to make a decision based on a shortcut such as "Anything chocolate is good."

Stress has also been shown to temper our willingness to suffer more in the short term in order to achieve a better long-term gain.[8] Higher levels of stress hormones circulating in the brain reduce the normal release of dopamine, the neurotransmitter that signals feelings of reward or pleasure,[9] and these lower dopamine levels seem to change the way we evaluate cost-benefit trade-offs. Effort seems harder, increasing the perceived cost of a particular option and reducing motivation to work for the promised benefit. Instead, we are more apt to favor the expedient choice. ("It's too hard to find an expert in my cancer, so I'll just go with the doctor I've already met.")

Over time, we find it harder to concentrate, and we begin to belabor decisions, becoming indecisive and more anxious about committing. This is particularly challenging if we are making a series of decisions, each one of which feels progressively harder, leaving us increasingly depleted and less able to make the next one. Remember taking standardized tests in school? The questions always seemed harder by the time we got to the end of the test, in large part because we suffered from decision fatigue. It turns out that brains, like muscles, get tired from an extensive workout and need refueling. Rest and a recovery snack help with mental as well as physical fitness.

While each of us might have a different way of reaching

what we consider a good decision, we can all agree that making choices about our care in the heat of the moment is hard. There is no way to know all the answers or understand with certainty what our expectations for "best outcomes" should be. But being aware of our innate tendencies and the impact of stress on the process can help make things a little easier.

Given the taxing nature of complex decision-making, be sure to give your brain the glucose it needs to make the hard decisions. Eat a cookie, take a nap, or better still, sleep on it—turns out, that's really good advice. You can also try reducing your stress and putting yourself into a good mood. Take some deep breaths, go for a walk, watch a funny video, play with the dog, hug someone you love. All these will lower your stress hormones and help you engage more of your brain. Then, go make the best decision you can. You'll feel better with the decision behind you.

While no cancer decision is truly easy, situations that involve greater complexity and uncertainty are especially challenging and lead to delayed and belabored decisions. In addition to rare cancers, like Jane's, a number of other situations can increase the degree of difficulty, including multiple treatment protocol options, treatment that creates fertility issues or leads to reconstruction choices, the implications of genetic testing on additional surgery, and even the prospect of participating in clinical trials.

Zero Chance of a Baby

Fatima had a hard time coming to grips with her diagnosis of endometrial cancer at age thirty-six. In the middle of an internship that would lead to a medical assistant certification, she was used to being on the other side of the dialogue, not receiving scary information, so when her gynecologist told her the news, it took her a while to grasp the full impact of his pronouncement. But after getting opinions from two gynecological oncologists, the reality sank in. "My husband and I were trying to have kids, but both doctors said the best chance I had for getting rid of the cancer was to remove my entire reproductive system, which would mean zero chance of having a baby," she said.

It was a lot to absorb; not only was she facing a scary diagnosis and massive surgery, but treatment was going to radically change her life. If she spared her ovaries, there was a chance she could later harvest her eggs and find a surrogate to have her babies, but there was also a greater risk the cancer would come back. In addition to giving up the notion of conceiving her own children, Fatima had to accept the idea that the recommended surgery would throw her into instant menopause.

> I had a lot of anxiety about making the right decision. So much was going to change. But after talking with my husband and family, I decided I had to do what was best to survive. I scheduled the surgery and then it was like a train that was moving forward—the scans and the blood work and the pre-op clearance—I didn't have time to think about cancer anymore.

Leslie wasn't even in a steady relationship when she was confronted with the question of whether or not she wanted to preserve her fertility. Thirty-one and working as an administrator in a London university, she was sitting in the breast clinic waiting to hear the results of her biopsy when the doctor started asking questions.

> First, he asked if I was on my own, then he asked if I had children, and if I wanted them. I told him I hadn't really decided, and he just continued saying, "Well, we have determined that you have cancer." It was surreal. I couldn't understand what this connection was between children and cancer. I was really quite resentful about that. I found it so maddening to be in a room and have to answer, while I'm in shock, do I want children? In the space of a week, I had to decide on a future plan that I really hadn't thought about.

Which Breast Is Best?

The options for reconstruction create a number of challenging decisions for breast cancer patients requiring mastectomies, or even some lumpectomies. Silicone or saline implants, tissue flap procedures, fat grafting, nipple/areola tattooing, and going flat are all options, depending on the size and location of the cancer, the extent of surgery to remove the cancer, and subsequent treatments needed, as well as patient preferences, health, breast size, and lifestyle considerations, not to mention insurance coverage. Surgical oncologists usually remove the tumor, while plastic surgeons rebuild the breast, either at the time of the cancer surgery or at a later date. But figuring all this out requires extensive research and coordination. Patients have to get familiar with the options appropriate to their condition and prioritize a set of abstract concepts, such as recovery time, risk of complications, and desired and likely future appearance.

When Noreen needed a biopsy for a lump on her breast, she knew it made sense to start thinking about the possibility of cancer but was unprepared for the deluge of decisions. "The doctor who did the biopsy in his office asked if I wanted him to be my surgeon before we even had the results back, and that really turned me off," she said. "I wasn't ready yet. Even though I was sure this wasn't going to be bad, I also had the sense that this wasn't really happening, that this wasn't really my life." Still numb from the news, she enlisted the help of friends to collect a number of recommendations, eventually making appointments with two breast surgeons. Then the hard work began.

> There were so many decisions and so many trade-offs for each one. One doctor thought a lumpectomy would do it; the other suggested a mastectomy, which, while more involved, was less frightening than the thought that a lumpectomy might not get it all.
>
> My husband was supportive of whatever, even going flat, but I felt reconstruction would make me more comfortable. And then there were more choices. My sister-in-law had had a double mastectomy with silicone implants that didn't serve her

well. They had to be taken out, and I didn't want to have to go back to the hospital again for more surgery. I thought I wanted a TRAM [transverse rectus abdominis muscle] flap procedure, but it's a very intense surgery and would take a toll on my body and mind.

The surgeon I ended up using took me through everything, from what the tests were showing to what she recommended, drawing pictures as she went. Her guidance helped a lot, but ultimately, I had to make the decision. It was hard to be rational at a time when I was so emotional.

Despite the challenges, Noreen was able to make her decisions and schedule surgery a month after her diagnosis, within the period most oncologists would think appropriate. Robin S. found she needed to stretch that to nearly two months in order to make the decisions she faced.

I was still in shock about my diagnosis when I met the first reconstruction surgeon, and really struggling with the idea of plastic surgery, which was antithetical to the natural way I lived my life. Everything in his office screamed "fake" and I had a hard time with that. By the time I met with the second reconstruction surgeon, I think I had a clearer sense of what I wanted, and he seemed patient with me as I made him answer the same questions over and over again. Eventually, I got comfortable enough to schedule surgery, but it took me a while to get there.

For Claire, a forty-year-old magazine editor and the mother of two young kids, it happened quickly, but not without a struggle. "It was the hardest decision I had to make, ever," she said. With a family history of breast cancer, her discovery of a lump when she was in the shower one morning prompted an urgent trip to the gynecologist, then scans that confirmed a malignancy.

> I felt so impotent. I asked the doctor what to do, but he said it was my decision. Every day for a week, I spoke with a different woman about her decision— did she have a lumpectomy or mastectomy? Did she do reconstruction? It was clearly so emotionally draining for them to tell me their stories, to go back and think about that time. I knew I didn't want to live in the constant state of "What's next?" even though there is always that possibility—it only takes one cell—so in the end, I told the surgeon to take both breasts and skip the reconstruction. I didn't ever want to feel that way again.

Stephanie was not so fortunate. A single mom with a busy life, full of kids and a job and caring for others, she ended up with six surgeries over a space of eighteen months. Her family's breast cancer history and ten years of comparative mammograms helped her move quickly from discovering a lump to having a diagnosis, but then things got complicated.

> When I saw the breast surgeon, she thought I could do just a lumpectomy, perhaps radiation. But the pathology report after surgery showed that they

hadn't gotten it all, and I had four kinds of cancerous cells in a single tumor, including aggressive pleomorphic cells. They would have to go back in to clear the margins.

When they went back in, they discovered my cancer was like a wagon wheel with spokes throughout my breast and they couldn't get it all. Meanwhile, it turns out they couldn't do radiation because I had had radio-frequency ablation to my heart for an electrical issue in the same area as my cancer. They sent me for chemo for five months, and then I had to decide on a single or bilateral mastectomy.

I worried about the pleomorphic cells and didn't want to have to go through all this again, so opted for the double, to be followed by reconstruction with implants. I had an issue with scar tissue, so I had to have another surgery before the implants could be placed and the reconstruction finished.

I'm a big rule follower, and I trusted my doctors, so I did what they told me to do. I wanted to understand it all and make the right decisions, but you don't know all the facts when you have to make your choices.

Too Many Facts

Not knowing all the facts is hard, but sometimes, knowing too many can add to the distress as well. Because of a family history with cancer, Terri was tested for her cancer gene (BRCA) status at age eighteen. She learned she was positive, and had a mammogram or breast magnetic resonance imaging (MRI) every six months thereafter.

> It was a curse. I spent my twenties waiting to get cancer and it affected every decision in my life. I really wanted to be a mother, to breastfeed, to have a normal life. So, when I got the diagnosis at age thirty, I was angry. I had to put my life on hold. If it had happened in my forties and I had already married and had kids, maybe I would have felt relief, but I was so young, just feeling some success in my job and nowhere near motherhood. They had been talking to me since my twenties about getting a prophylactic double mastectomy, but I didn't really understand how cancer worked and that it could have been prevented. So now, do I spend my thirties worrying about getting ovarian cancer, or do I have the surgery, which will ensure I never have kids but keeps me safe?

Brenda had the same quandary in reverse. Diagnosed with ovarian cancer at age fifty-eight, she had genetic testing as part of her follow-up care after surgery and chemotherapy. When she found out she was BRCA-positive, she had to make a choice.

> I realized I was a time bomb waiting to explode. I hated the idea of more surgery and knew how grueling recovery could be, but I scheduled a bilateral mastectomy as soon as I had recovered from the chemo. Even though it meant two major cancer surgeries in the space of a year, I knew it was the right decision. I couldn't relax until it was done.

ADVICE FROM THOSE WHO LEARNED IT THE HARD WAY

Making decisions under duress is never easy, and each of us has a different set of choices to make, a different set of unknowable outcomes, a different set of values underlying our preferences, and different approaches to making decisions. However, patients who have been through it offer some consistent advice. It starts with being well informed.

"Don't be afraid to get a second opinion," said Deborah. "Don't worry about insulting your doctor; just do it. You want to be sure you have the best information to make your decision." Rob agreed. "Don't go with what's thrown at you first," he said. "Take the time to investigate so you can be confident in your decision."

Making sure you really understand what the doctors have advised is also a consistent theme. "Go back to the doctor a couple of days after you've gotten the news to ask questions," said Leslie. "It empowers you, and helps you make it your decision, not theirs." Jane M. agreed. "Ask lots of questions," she said. "We're not experts, and the doctors and nurses are so focused on the disease it may not occur to them to reassure us about or even anticipate the things we worry about."

Given the stressfulness of the decisions, many people also find that having company through the process is helpful. "Bring someone to all your appointments who can take notes," said Claire. "You can't rely on your memory when it's time to make a decision—there's too much you don't hear." Elyse had similar insights. "Don't go to any appointment alone," she stressed. "You never know when you might get new crappy news. Allow yourself to accept support from others, even if you are always independent."

But perhaps the best advice is to recognize that it is *your* decision, and not up to the doctor or family members or friends. As Cass put it, "Do your research, ask a lot of questions, get advice from others, and then make the decision that feels comfortable to you. You are the one who has to live with it." Recognizing how challenging the process is and that none of us can make the perfect decision is key. "At some point, you have to trust that you're making the best decision you can with the information you have and just forgive yourself for any mistakes," said Catherine. "Be gentle and loving and patient with yourself. It's an incredibly intense time." Or, as Robin A. said, "We make decisions the best we can; then we make them right or wrong by the way we live them. So make your decision, then make it work."

SIDEBAR: SHAPING COMMUNICATIONS TO MEET PATIENTS' NEEDS

A good doctor will try to adjust communication with a patient to offer a balance of information and encouragement at a challenging time, particularly when trying to make important healthcare decisions. But this is not always an easy task, even for seasoned professionals. **Dr. Peter Dottino, former director of gynecologic oncology at Mount Sinai Health System in New York** where he continues as **clinical gynecologic oncologist and surgeon, and professor of obstetrics, gynecology, and reproductive science,** has treated thousands of patients in thirty-five years of practice, describes his thought process and how to get what you need from a conversation with your doctor.

How do you communicate with patients to reduce their anxiety?

I try to demystify the disease and treatment based on what the patient needs to know, wants to hear, and can handle. The first question all patients want answered is, "Am I going to die from this?" I try to address that in the first few moments we're together so that I can defuse the stress. It's very hard for patients to hear anything else I have to say if they are still focused on that question.

continued

What do you try to cover in that first meeting with a patient?

Patients come to me because they have been told to find a cancer surgeon, but I don't know up front what else they have been told—what they know about their condition. I want to make sure they leave my office with a clear understanding of their diagnosis, the recommended treatment plan, and their prognosis. I try to make my explanations as straightforward as I can, generally going through the information once, writing things down for the patients, and suggesting they think about it and call me with questions or come back again if they want to talk more.

How do you adjust your communication to meet the needs of each patient?

Patients are dealing with a lot of emotion when they come to see me. Even though they already know they have cancer and their initial shock has passed, it can take a while to own it—to accept that you are a cancer patient. Unfortunately, most patients know someone who has had cancer, and their understanding of *that* cancer experience becomes the benchmark for how they view their own, even if it's totally irrelevant. I have to pick up cues from patients I've just met about their assumptions and anxiety levels and what they are able to take in, and help them get beyond the stigma and fear to see that there are so many options, that things really aren't as bad as they fear.

What clues do you listen for in speaking with a patient?

I can tell a lot about how patients are doing and how much they have understood in the conversation by the questions they ask. Sometimes I have to answer the same question multiple times as the patient comes to terms with what she has been told. If her anxiety prevents her from hearing important information, I try to come at it from a different angle, present it in a different way. Once a patient is asking about next steps, I know she is ready to move into survival mode, to do what needs to be done. But not everyone can get there in a single meeting. That's why written notes are so important.

What can patients do to help themselves in this process?

There are several things patients can do that make it easier for themselves and their doctors in the early meetings. The first is to think about the important things that will help guide your decision. What are your biggest concerns? What are your personal priorities? Some people like to do a lot of research, some don't want to know anything a doctor hasn't told them personally, and I'm fine with either. But if you are going to research your cancer, do it on sites published by reputable medical institutions; don't go reading a bunch of blog posts that will elevate your anxiety.

Do come with a written list of questions you want answered so you can walk out of the visit with the answers

continued

you need. And, most importantly, bring someone along on those first few visits—someone who can take notes and help keep track of questions to be answered. There is so much to absorb at a time when you are under so much stress, it's best if someone is writing it all down so you can think about it again later. But please don't bring the whole family. It's hard for the patient—and for the doctor—if too many people are involved.

Ultimately, the decision rests with the patient, but I can offer as much guidance and assistance as a patient wants. The art is to figure out what will best support the patient when she is struggling to understand that herself.

LIFE OUT OF BALANCE: SUBMITTING TO CARE

"Start by doing what's necessary; then do what's possible; and suddenly you are doing the impossible."

—*Francis of Assisi*

Beginning cancer treatment, whatever the first step might be, often brings a sense of relief; you know that, finally, someone will be dealing with the cancer that has kept you sleepless for so many nights. But that relief is also tinged with anxiety and fear. Like stepping over the edge into an abyss, you are headed into the unknown: "What exactly is going to happen to my body when they start?" "What will they discover when they cut me open?" "How will I respond to chemo?" "Will radiation cause a burn?" "Will I be able to tolerate immunotherapy?" With more than five hundred varieties and combinations of therapies and the accelerating rate at which new medications are being approved by the U.S. Food and Drug Administration (FDA),[1] there can be no blanket statement about the likely side effects of cancer treatment. Add to that the unpredictable and individualized responses we all have to medications of any sort, and it can be hard to anticipate what you might feel.

Advances in how treatment is delivered have taken some of the sting out of it for many patients. Laparoscopy, which uses multiple small incisions and a miniature camera to allow the surgeon to see inside the patient without making a large incision, has become the preferred method for many cancer surgeries, reducing recovery times and the pain of surgery.[2] The addition of anti-nausea medication, antihistamines, and steroids to chemo infusions has lessened the propensity for vomiting and other extreme responses. Reduced and targeted radiation has decreased the frequency of radiation burns and adverse effects. Immunotherapies, which stimulate the patient's own immune cells to recognize and fight cancer cells, and targeted therapies, which work by destroying cells with specific cancerous mutations, cause few or no side effects for some lucky patients. Still, we are a long way from having the precision medicine of the future, where doctors will be able to sequence the DNA of every patient's healthy and cancerous cells to determine exactly which remedy will provide the cure with the least misery, and most of us still will undergo at least one of the more toxic treatments.

Uncertainty about the coming experience, coupled with continued anxiety about the efficacy of treatment and our prospects for recovery, makes this a stressful time for many cancer patients. While loved ones and medical experts try to reassure us that we will get through, often what we feel is a sense of existential dread, and the isolation that comes with believing we are alone in our fears. As Jane M. said, "It would be very difficult for anyone who isn't going through it to understand."

Carl echoed that sentiment. When he found a clinical trial to treat his "incurable" melanoma, he was relieved but terrified. "No one was saying that the odds were good. There were so few of us, and everyone was so sick. I mostly confided in my wife. But I was so needy, I wasn't sure I could share my fears even with her and felt so isolated."

An Emotional Black Hole

A filmmaker and TV producer, thirty-six-year-old Elyse had a bump on her eye socket and persistent fatigue that she dismissed as the inevitability of motherhood. But when the bump finally led her to an eye doctor who said the mass showed pre-lymphoma cells, she knew she was in for a ride. Additional testing with a lymphoma specialist showed she had cancer throughout her body—stage 4 lymphoma.

> When they started me on a monthlong course of immunotherapy, they were not very optimistic, and sitting there in the infusion suite with people who were so much sicker than me, I felt guilty that I was so scared. It was an emotional black hole.
>
> I'm a pretty private person and don't include everyone in my own moments of vulnerability, so I just tucked away my fear and didn't know what to do with it. People think that a diagnosis exists in a

vacuum, but it's a deep, deep grief that you weave into your daily life as you go through treatment and recovery—it's a continuum. There is this incredible sense of vulnerability that comes from understanding that your body—the body that you have counted on and taken for granted—has betrayed you, and you have to grieve for that. No matter how much support you have or don't have, you're the one who has to go through it. That's the isolation.

Newly awakened to this vulnerability, we see how our bodies can betray us, how cancer can hide, how doctors can overlook things, and how medicine can fail. This new understanding makes it hard to relax, even as we are hopeful about treatment. "No one tells you that you can still live through cancer and treatment," said Nickie, diagnosed with multiple myeloma a year after successful surgery for pancreatic cancer. "If you assume you're going to die, you get focused on dying rather than living, and that makes you feel isolated. You have to do more about the living part of your life." But for a lot of patients, that's hard.

Solace from the Ubiquity of Cancer

Not everyone experiences a sense of isolation. Given that nearly 40 percent of us will receive a cancer diagnosis at some point in our lives,[3] it's hard not to know someone who is going through or has gone through the experience. This is particularly true of breast cancer. One in eight women gets breast cancer, and because of earlier detection and better treatment plans, most survive. While that's great news for the physical health of those with a new diagnosis, it also eases the emotional experience for many by reducing the sense of isolation. That was certainly the case for Teresa, a former book editor, who was sixty-seven years old when she got the news that she had advanced breast cancer.

> I never felt isolated. I had family members who had had breast cancer and had a friend with colon cancer who had been through chemo, and a friend going through treatment for bone cancer at the same time I was receiving my treatment. Even being in a room for treatment with other cancer patients at the cancer center sort of normalized it. All my cousins with breast cancer were fine. That reinforced my belief that this was going to work—that treatment would eliminate the cancer, and I was going to survive.

Many patients also struggle with relinquishing control when they start treatment—control over their schedules, their bodies, their minds, their lives. However you may have lived before your diagnosis, no matter how much or how little power you had to set your own schedule, rule your own life, and plan your days, cancer demands your full attention and cancer treatment takes over your life. Surgery happens when the doctor can squeeze you in; radiation happens every day. Infusions occur on a fixed schedule mandated by the rigors of the particular protocol and the normal reproductive cycle of human blood cells. Work commitments, family schedules, vacation plans—everything goes out the window as you follow the dictates of a new boss. And even after you have your treatment schedule in place, don't put anything on your calendar in permanent ink! The calendar may dictate when you have to be where for treatment, but how long it will take and how you will respond and what you can and can't do on any given day are all up for grabs. Letting go of control is one more thing patients have to do. Just as you suspend your need to read the map when Google says to take the next right, you have to be willing to follow directions, do as you are told, and try not to deviate from the prescribed path.

"You can't control cancer, but you want to control something," said Nancy H., fifty-six years old when she had surgery for ovarian cancer. "That sense of loss of control is horrible. When I woke up in the hospital and discovered that my daughter had silenced my phone so I wouldn't be disturbed, I was upset. I understood why she did it, but it felt like one more thing out of my control."

Melanie, a fifty-year-old entrepreneur, was determined to maintain control over her breast cancer experience, even in the face of reality. "I'm a control freak, and it didn't dawn on me that I wasn't in charge," she said. "Once I realized a mastectomy was nonnegotiable, I switched my focus to reconstruction options, and then tried to get control over treatment. I told the oncologist that I was available to start chemo in January (three months away). She said, 'Are you crazy? You are going to start now.'"

Jane M. also was used to being in control—in the office, when kayaking, and in her life. She found learning to roll with it through cancer difficult after decades of self-determination.

> There is always uncertainty in your life, more than
> you recognize, because of the proverbial truck that

could come out of nowhere and plow into you, but you manage to assume you have a degree of control that you really don't. You live your life thinking, "If I do this, it will advance my career; we can plan a vacation here, and do this then." You build an entire structure around things that you think are certainties. But when cancer comes along, it blows that all up, and all of a sudden, you deal with uncertainty on a regular basis. Eventually, you stop fighting; it is what it is. It's wasted energy to try to build on quicksand, and you don't have that energy to waste.

Because losing control over life can be so disorienting, some patients fight the loss by micromanaging other aspects of their care. As Jane said, "There are certain things you need to be mellow about. If you get a biopsy, you have to wait a week to learn the results. There is nothing you can do about that and you just need to accept it. But if you call someone to get an appointment and that person doesn't call back, you can do something about that. I'm still type A in those situations."

Teresa knew she couldn't control the cancer, but she was used to managing against a deadline, so she did her best to direct the rest.

Once I had started, my objective was to just get through this. I would be at the mercy of the treatment and knew that my life was about to be out of control in very important ways. Treatment was once a week and I knew my start time, but what about the end time? How would I feel? Side effects? Would it work? That would be my life for five months, so I took control of everything I could. I arranged transportation to get to and from treatment, started working out intensely, learned what I could about diet and potential intestinal issues. It wasn't much, but it made me feel better about the stuff I couldn't control.

Stella, a thirty-two-year-old advertising and marketing entrepreneur, was used to breaking the rules. So when she got her diagnosis of breast cancer, she questioned her doctor's advice to follow surgery with chemotherapy and investigated alternatives to make her own treatment plan.

You feel out of control because you have to do so many things. First a lumpectomy, then a port, then chemo. People are telling you what you have to do, and you just do it. The doctor wanted to schedule the lumpectomy for a week after my diagnosis and I felt it was too fast. Then I met a woman who told me about insulin potentiated therapy (IPT), which uses insulin to hypersensitize cancer cells to the chemo toxins and reduces the dose of chemo needed with each infusion. This seemed like a better option to me. If you are going to be putting your body through so much, why not make it a little better? How can your body recover from all that poison if you don't also help it? I postponed the surgery for two weeks and said I would do the IPT instead of regular chemo. I felt like I had a little bit of control over what my journey was going to be.

(Because there were no studies published in leading medical journals demonstrating the effectiveness of IPT compared to standard chemotherapy, Stella's doctor advised against her decision and for five years encouraged her to get traditional chemo. Eventually, he stopped insisting; today, ten years after her surgery with no recurrence, he just tells her to keep doing whatever it is she is doing, because it seems to be working for her.)

Elyse was less radical in her approach to taking charge; she followed her doctor's orders on chemotherapy but put her own unique stamp on the process. "What really changed the experience for me," she said, "was taking my camera. It created a completely different effect. I felt in control. It was a creative project and allowed me to be a little bit in a professional mode, rather than the victim, as I watched them violate me with a needle each time. I hate needles. But I have always felt safe and calm and confident behind the camera; bringing my camera to treatment was a way of taking back a little of the power of the experience."

A Haunting Disease

While dealing with the loss of control over their lives, patients also struggle with fear and anxiety, which never quite go away. As Mark said of his liver cancer, diagnosed when he was sixty, two years after his open-heart surgery, "Cancer is scarier than heart disease, because everyone knows that none of the treatments are going to be fun. Plus, heart disease is a quick fix—they operate and then you're well again. At least it was for me after my bypass. It's not like it's going to come back. But cancer is a haunting disease, and you never know if the treatment is going to work."

Steve, who had had testicular cancer more than twenty-five years before a diagnosis of colon cancer at age fifty-five, agreed. "They told me at the time that I was predisposed to getting another cancer. Now I'm terrified of it coming back yet again. When I go for treatment, I see that I'm one of the younger patients in the infusion center. The idea that it could come back when I am older and don't have the strength to fight it is tough. I don't want to be a burden to someone when I'm seventy or eighty years old."

Mary R. had been reassured that she would be fine when she started treatment for her Hodgkin's lymphoma. "Relapse rates are low, and chemo outcomes are pretty good," she said. "But on the first day, they handed me a fifty-page list of all the symptoms I might have. That freaked me out. How many people get these symptoms, and what do people do about it? My anxiety about the disease was bad enough, but worrying about all these side effects was overwhelming."

And the physical side effects of treatment are definitely real. Recovering from surgery is hard. It can take weeks to shake the last of the anesthesia out of one's system. And depending on what has been cut from where, incisional pain and adjusting to organs having been rearranged can take months. The painkillers that are offered bring their own delights: usually constipation that is even harder to deal with when you have chest or abdominal stitches, as well as the threat of addiction and rebound pain.

When nonsurgical therapy starts, nausea and fatigue are the most common side effects, but depending on the treatment, and whether it is infused into the circulatory system, aimed at or pumped right into an affected area of the body, or swallowed in the form of pills, all sorts of other effects may be felt.

Mark's liver cancer was treated with chemoembolization, which meant delivering the chemo directly to his liver via a catheter inserted in his femoral artery. "Even though they gave me drugs during the procedure, I always felt pain afterward from the incision, and a sharp pain where they treated the cancer. My organs felt invaded. Plus, I was tired, couldn't eat much, and lost my sense of taste—pizza tasted the same as the cardboard box it came in. But two weeks later, it was over, and I just had to wait until the next one."

Nancy H. was well past menopause when she had her ovaries removed, but that didn't stop her from going through menopause all over again. "I wasn't really symptomatic with menopause, but definitely was after surgery," she said. "I wasn't expecting that, but you get a little something from your ovaries even after they have stopped releasing eggs. On top of that, they threw chemo at me. I lost my hair, gained thirty pounds despite being nauseated, was tired all the time, and had neuropathy in my feet, dry skin, and chemo brain that ten years later still affects my ability to think."

Stephanie wasn't expecting to have chemotherapy or any follow-up care when she went in for a lumpectomy the first time. But when the pathology report showed a more complicated picture, with four different types of cancer, she was started on chemo in anticipation of a mastectomy down the road. "A lot of folks have surgery and then go into chemo. Having it the other way meant that when they removed the breast tissue, we could see from the pathology report that the chemo had worked. That was positive, but I went to surgery with no hair, and feeling so vulnerable. That whole process was hard, and even though it is three years later, my hair is still not what it was. I have a lot of spots where the hair just never regrew."

In addition to the usual side effects of chemo, such as nausea, fatigue, hair loss, and neuropathy, Teresa's treatment gave her palmar-plantar erythrodysesthesia, commonly called hand-foot syndrome, a rare side effect in which the chemo leaks from the capillaries of the fingers and toes. "Blood would accumulate under my fingernails and be very painful," said Teresa. "The oncologist paid no attention to it, but when it was very bad, I would cry in the treatment chair and the nurses would offer all kinds of suggestions. Eventually, I saw my surgeon, who lanced my thumbs to let the blood out and put me in the hospital for about two days on antibiotics while they continued with the treatment plan."

Jennifer had a type of chemo for her ovarian cancer called hyperthermic intraperitoneal chemotherapy (HIPEC), essentially a hot chemo bath circulating through her abdomen. "Every cell of my body screamed in agony and hurt so bad," she said. "Nothing tasted good, food was horrid, and the whole first week was just excruciating. But I had declared that chemo wouldn't defeat me, so I didn't stay in bed. I sat in my chair a lot, but not bed!"

Ann F. found that radiation made her more tired than chemo did. "I didn't have the energy to stand on the bus going to and from treatment, but it was hard to get a seat," she said. "One time, I cried when no one would offer me theirs. And my breast burned. It was as red as an apple. I tried all kinds of lotions, but the discoloration and pain lasted a really long time."

Whatever the cancer treatment, these physical changes, particularly pain and inflammation, cause additional physical and emotional stress and affect brain chemistry. And these chemical changes can leave us feeling attacked on all sides, increasing our vulnerability at what is already a very emotional time.

SCIENCE SIDEBAR: THE CHEMISTRY EXPERIMENT IN YOUR BRAIN

A variety of forces gang up on us during cancer treatment, causing changes in the brain and leading to increased emotional volatility and variability. The disease itself; surgery; the anesthesia from surgery; the increased cortisol from stress and constant pain, not to mention the synthetic cortisol—prednisone or dexamethasone—we may be taking as part of treatment; hormonal changes as a result of surgery and treatment; and chemo/immunotherapy drugs all contribute to changes in our emotional response.

One of the key drivers of this increased emotional variability is a class of proteins called cytokines, which our bodies produce to help cells in our immune systems communicate and coordinate to fight threats. There are pro-inflammation cytokines and anti-inflammation cytokines that work together to initiate an immune response when a threat is perceived, and resolve it when the threat has passed. Get a paper cut, and pro-inflammation cytokines are released to tell your body to bring white blood cells and platelets to the site to heal the wound. A virus, too much exercise, pollen—there are lots of ways to trigger an immune response, and they all involve pro-inflammatory cytokines. The anti-inflammatory cytokines kick in when the cut is healed, the virus eradicated, the muscles repaired. It is the balance of the two classes of cytokines that keeps an immune system healthy, and it's the imbalance that leads to autoimmune diseases such as allergies and rheumatoid arthritis. Somehow, the signal to shut

continued

down the inflammation doesn't get through, and we stay inflamed.

There is always some cytokine activity going on in the body; the bigger the threat, the greater the activity. Not surprisingly, cancer is perceived by the body as a threat and causes pro-inflammatory cytokines to be released, as does the stress we feel as a result of having cancer. Double whammy. And if a paper cut can release cytokines, just imagine what surgery can do. Radiation? Check. Chemotherapy? Check. Even the successful outcome of treatment, the death of cancer cells, increases cytokines. We are swimming in pro-inflammatory cytokines as we start cancer treatment.

But cytokines are not all bad. They also are used to help fight cancer. Some immunotherapy treatments harness the natural power of specific cytokines to regulate immune response: interleukin 2, which is produced by the body to help fight infection, and interferon-alpha, which helps fight off viruses and bacteria. These cytokines are infused like chemo to stimulate antibodies and attack unhealthy cells. But they do come with nasty side effects.

While doing their thing in our bodies, cytokines also affect the brain. One way they do this is by interfering with the normal functioning of the prefrontal cortex (the rational part of the brain), allowing the limbic system (the emotional part of the brain) to rule the day. In the presence of elevated cytokines, the brain signals the body to behave as if it's sick, leading to fatigue and flu-like symptoms that drive us back to bed when the rational part of the brain might otherwise encourage us to get up and go for a walk. We feel less motivated to do anything, and more tearful and dependent. This sickness behavior is a good thing if we have a fever, helping us rest and get the care from others we need to recover from the threat. But it is less productive when what we are facing is emotional stress—hiding under the covers doesn't help us deal with the anxiety caused by a boss who is unrelenting in his criticism. So when we get a devastating diagnosis, it's not just that we are tired and mopey because we have cancer, but also that our cytokines are in overdrive and keep telling us to shut down. Some of that is good—after all, our bodies are working hard at recovery—but it can be too much of a good thing when we don't bounce back after surgery and treatment.

Experts now think that interference with the normal functioning of the prefrontal cortex also contributes to emotional volatility in cancer, and especially to depression. And depression is one of the major side effects of pro-inflammatory cytokine interferon therapy.[4] The inflammatory response also suppresses the release of dopamine, the natural reward hormone, which decreases motivation and arousal while increasing sensitivity to negative input from the environment. We become hypervigilant and protective against attack,[5] which feeds into anxiety about the disease and about prognosis. We're more aware of every physical sensation and we assume it's related to the cancer. Increased anxiety leads to increased cytokines and makes us more likely to skip that walk when exercise might actually help reduce the inflammation and put those cytokines back in balance. It's a downward spiral of inflammation and

continued

angst. No wonder it can be hard to get on with life while fighting cancer!

A key variable in this cytokine response is perceived control over stress.[6] When a stress is predictable and we can control it, we learn to manage it—our brains become wired for dealing with that particular stress and it no longer causes an automatic inflammatory response. (Remember those firefighters in chapter 2?) But when a stress is perceived as uncontrollable, as in cancer, look out. That's when our bodies and brains become awash with cytokines.

As with most things having to do with emotions and the brain, each of us responds to inflammatory cytokines differently. Genetic predisposition and prior stress exposure, as well as body mass index, age, and gender (women are more likely than men to be sensitive to the behavioral effects of inflammation), play roles in how our systems respond to inflammation and the behavioral symptoms we experience, creating tremendous variations in our tendencies toward depression, irritable anger, poor appetite, and fatigue. And because cytokines also influence other neurotransmitters, such as serotonin, norepinephrine, and the hormone that kicks off the stress reaction, corticotrophin-releasing hormone, it can be hard to predict how any of us is going to feel. Suffice it to say, there is a chemistry experiment going on in there, making emotions run high.

And speaking of hormones: testosterone and estrogen, which we all have in varying amounts regardless of age or gender, take a beating with cancer. Surgery that removes any organs that produce or are receptive to hormones has an obvious impact, but so do stress and many treatments, such as estrogen or androgen suppression, that alter our baseline hormone levels and their natural fluctuations. Estrogen helps us manage fear and stress. Higher levels of estrogen increase physical and emotional resiliency. Sudden withdrawal of estrogen (as in premenstrual syndrome, postpartum depression, surgical removal of ovaries, or medical estrogen suppression) increases anxiety. Meanwhile, stress shuts down testosterone production, reducing our energy and stamina. And cortisol, either natural or in the synthetic form of prednisone or dexamethasone, messes around with both.

Many of these factors also affect sleep patterns, which in turn affect emotions. Disrupted sleep is frequently associated with depression, anxiety, and PTSD in a chicken-and-egg relationship that is difficult to sort out but often builds.[7] We are anxious because we are dealing with stress; the anxiety makes it difficult to sleep. Sleep disruptions throw off our natural cortisol cycles, making it harder for the prefrontal cortex to do its job, and we become more susceptible to our emotions, feeling more anxious, which makes it difficult to sleep.

In addition to this chemically induced emotional volatility, we often begin to struggle with cognitive changes. As we have seen, stress itself can inhibit normal thinking patterns, making us hyperfocused on the threat but unable to concentrate on just about everything else. And by interfering with the normal function of the prefrontal cortex, cytokines also affect memory, learning, and attention. Meanwhile,

continued

treatment itself, particularly chemotherapy, has been shown to interfere with thinking ability in direct and indirect ways. While this is not a universal experience, many patients—as many as 75 percent of those with breast cancer[8]—have cognitive changes while undergoing treatment. Whether it's called "cancer-related cognitive impairment" or "chemo-related cognitive dysfunction" or just plain "chemo brain," there is something going on we don't fully understand. Scientists think that cytokines are a contributing factor, but they also are exploring whether chemo and other treatments alter cognition by increasing cellular damage, driving changes in memory formation and learning. Increased oxidative stress, a normal side effect of metabolism that is usually kept in check by a healthy lifestyle, is another possible cause, as is the chance that chemo reprograms the way we produce new cells and synapses in the brain and alters the natural life span of brain cells.

Who among us will experience chemo brain and how noticeable it will be are influenced by a variety of factors: the type of treatment received, the degree to which we are already taxing our brains, genetics, age at time of treatment, and general health.[9] There is a lot of research on the effect, but few clear answers, particularly because it is such a difficult thing to measure and test. In the meantime, it is one more insult many patients must endure and contributes to the emotional response they have to the disease. The good news is that most chemo brain effects dissipate in one to two years, although that is a frustratingly long time.

It is common to experience emotional and cognitive changes during treatment. This is unsettling on many levels, but part of the problem is that cancer challenges us to

> reverse our thinking about health and health care. With most ailments, we have symptoms, we see a doctor for treatment, and we start to feel better. With cancer, often we feel fine until we get a diagnosis, the doctor gives us treatment, and we feel miserable physically, mentally, and emotionally. This is the misery phase, and few of us escape without some suffering. It does pass, maybe not fast enough, but it does.

Many patients have surprising responses to starting treatment. Jake found that he became a particularly aggressive driver when he was taking prednisone as part of his lymphoma chemo treatments, and Maria feared for her life when the prednisone her husband was taking as part of his treatment for multiple myeloma led to a severe psychotic episode while he was driving on a highway. Flu-like symptoms from breast cancer chemo kept Jillian in bed for a few days with each treatment, but then that would change. "The steroids made my skin look amazing and I felt fabulous," she said. Deborah found that treatment for her ovarian cancer made her agitated and sleep nearly impossible. "I was restless and had back pain and headaches and a rash—it just kind of wears you out," she said. Aparna also found the whole thing emotionally draining and was depressed and weepy throughout treatment. "The fear kept me frozen, deeply scared, and devoid of hope," she said. Shelley was surprised by the overwhelming fatigue that radiation for her breast cancer brought on. Every day for five weeks, the fatigue increased until it seemed it would swallow her whole, and then it was done.

ADVICE FROM THOSE WHO LEARNED IT THE HARD WAY

Starting treatment is an unsettling time as the body and brain go through many changes. While each of us is likely to respond to those changes in ways specific to our treatment and our own bodies, patients who have been there recommend some consistent approaches for getting through the first few weeks, starting with recognizing your strengths and limitations. Jane M. suggests that you treat the good days as if nothing had happened. "But on the bad days," she said, "you just cope the best you can. You dial back a little on your expectations of yourself and try to do some of what you used to do, but not all." Jennifer advised friends with cancer not to let it take over their lives. "Cancer doesn't define you," she said. "You are not just cancer; you're still who you were before your diagnosis." And Teresa said, "Control what you can, because so much is out of control. You'll feel better about life if you can find something that you can be in charge of."

Sometimes learning a little more can be beneficial. Ask questions. Talk to those who have been there. Steve reminded friends who were fighting cancer to talk to the nursing staff. "You'll get more answers from the nurses, and they have a caring instinct. They watch people struggling with the side effects of chemo and radiation all the time and have so many good ideas for how to deal with it all." Brian recommended talking to fellow sufferers. "Check in with support groups, even if they are online," he said. "It is so helpful to hear from others who have been there and know—who can say, 'Oh, yeah, that's perfectly normal.'"

But remember, you also need physical support to get through the treatment and the rest of daily life. Christina suggested building a network of people who can pitch in. "It is so important to have a support system in place and to use it. I never used to ask for help, but now I say 'Sure, I would love that' if someone offers to help. 'Thank you so much for doing that for me.' It helps them too. They are not going to heal you, as much as they might want to wave a magic wand, but they want to help. And they're doing little things for you that represent a big help when you are fatigued and overwhelmed. It makes you both feel better."

Trying to maintain some perspective during this particularly volatile phase is also important. Survivors generally agree that, as hard as it may be, taking things one step at a time and trying not to get overwhelmed by the big picture are good pieces of advice. As Susie said, "The best way to eat an elephant is one bite at a time. I think Ann Landers suggested that way back when, but it's great advice for dealing with cancer!" Or, as Lulu put it, "It's like being a boxer in a match. Every step is like a punch. It doesn't matter how that one landed because you have to be ready for the next one. You are in it for the victory, not the single blow."

Anne recommended being a "joy catcher." "Take strength from the small things around you," she said. "It helps you cope with the big thing, cancer." Bob agreed. "You can't change that you have cancer," he said. "You have to just accept it and keep moving forward. Finding optimism is really important. So put a smile on your face, have faith, and just put one foot in front of the other. Sometimes that's easier said than done, but that's the goal."

SIDEBAR: COPING STYLES

Each of us has our own inner strengths to draw on when facing challenges, and coping mechanisms that have been effective in reducing stress in the past will most likely work when dealing with cancer. But finding resilience through the ongoing ordeal may require trying new strategies and finding abilities we never knew we had. There are many ways to cope in a time of crisis, and no single "right" way.

Personality influences how we respond to challenges. For example, people who tend to be optimistic in outlook in general may experience less stress and avoid anticipating the worst. They cope with a problem by **facing it head-on** in an attempt to master it. People who tend to be pessimistic or anxiously cautious often cope by **letting off steam**, and sometimes find it hard to manage their own anxiety or distress. They often rely on **external support** to help them cope with distress. Some of us don't like ambiguity and want to solve problems right away; others need more time to adjust to a new reality. Some gather information; others prefer not to know. Some strive for independence; others rely on those around them. Denial, distractions, humor, prayer, exercise—all are valid if they work for you. And what works one day might not work the next, so it's good to have a few other approaches to fall back on.

Coping by Doing

There are two broad approaches we can take to help us cope—we can change what we *do* in response to a stressful situation, and we can change the way we *think* about it. Often, what we do can also influence how we think. A classic example is **sleep**. Getting a good night's rest helps us function better the next day, which allows us to do a better job of solving problems. But it is a physical thing that we do to help us cope. Similarly, **exercise** releases endorphins, which create a sense of well-being that can last for hours. When the fatigue of cancer sets in, it's hard to imagine going for a run or climbing a hill, but even a short walk can help. Sometimes as little as ten minutes, preferably outside on a sunny day, is all you need. Gardening, housework, sports, and more formal exercise routines can all help. They may even improve your sleep. Watching your **diet** to be sure you are feeding your brain and keeping your body healthy while minimizing nicotine, caffeine, and alcohol can also help provide clarity.

Other things we can do to help us cope include **being social**, **defining a purpose**, **expressing gratitude**, and laughing or **using humor**. By nature, we are social creatures and tend to thrive when we are close to other people, be they family, friends, or colleagues. And the more social connections we have, the more resilient we seem to be. For instance, Ted fell apart when he had to deal with cancer treatment. Always a pessimist, he could see only the way the disease was going to take over his life. A self-described "basket case," he relied heavily on his wife—his primary social connection—and talked with her about his fears. She reminded him that this was not the first crisis he had faced and helped him find information from knowledgeable friends to allay his concerns. While he couldn't imagine going through it without her, he was fortunate enough not to have to.

continued

Defining a **sense of purpose,** whether grand or quotidian, can help you focus your energy in a positive way. Maybe you want to be of service to others while you deal with your stress, or maybe you just want to make sure you put a healthy meal on the table regularly. Being able to use your unique combination of strengths and talents can contribute to feelings of accomplishment and overall well-being.

Similarly, taking time to reflect on the positive side of things and finding ways to express **gratitude** can help us shift our thought patterns. Some people find that keeping a journal, writing down every week the things that they are grateful for, no matter how small, helps them stay in the moment and release their anxiety. It can also help you see your current situation in balance with your life as a whole, which often gets pushed aside when you're overwhelmed by a crisis.

Using **humor** or a lighter perspective in dealing with a challenging situation is another effective way to reduce stress. While there is nothing funny about having cancer, there is well-documented evidence that laughter actually lowers the level of stress hormones and helps diffuse negative emotions. Betsy put humor to work for her as she explained to friends how losing her hair gave her back years of life and would facilitate an early retirement—all the time spent washing and drying her hair added up to months, and the money she saved on haircuts, color touch-ups, and multiple hair products added up to a small fortune. This unusual twist allowed her to make the best of a bad situation and had the extra benefit of putting her family and friends at ease. As hard as it was to face her own bald head in the mirror, she didn't want to deal with other people's reactions and found that shared laughter over the absurdity of it all reduced their discomfort and hers while contributing to greater closeness.

Coping by Thinking

The flip side of the "doing" approach is the "thinking" approach—using what we know about ourselves to help us think through and manage the crisis. **Problem-solving, prioritizing,** and **avoiding unnecessary stressors** help us deal with the big one staring us in the face. While we can't eliminate the cancer stress, are there other worries and responsibilities we can reduce or eliminate to allow us to cope better? Can we reframe the problem or adjust our standards to make things more manageable?

Any problem-solving approach starts by clearly identifying the problem, brainstorming to generate a list of possible solutions, evaluating the pros and cons of each, and choosing the option that is most rewarding and feasible. For example, Tom was up for a promotion when he got his diagnosis, and he was determined not to let anything get in the way of that. Self-sufficient and a planner by nature, to solve this problem he asked his doctor if there were a way to schedule care around his work obligations, including a series of presentations he had to prepare and deliver. By collaborating with his doctor on a treatment schedule, he was able to fit in his work on the down days of treatment and still feel as if he were in control of his life.

continued

Many patients find that trying to maintain a "normal" routine while adding in the demands of treatment is overwhelming. Their problem-solving approach is often **prioritization** to make best use of limited energy. One way to prioritize is by type of task, delegating those that others could do. For instance, Beth was overwhelmed with care for her young children while undergoing chemo. She asked other family members to take her children to and from school during the weeks following treatments. Relinquishing this simple responsibility relieved some of her distress and allowed her to get the rest she needed. Asking friends to drop off dinner three days a week, or explaining to your boss why you want to involve a teammate to support you in the big project you were just assigned, and accepting that the lawn will not get mowed every week are all ways of reducing stress to preserve energy for the main event. Remembering that this change is temporary may help take the sting out of stepping away from some obligations, while allowing friends and family to help you can strengthen those social ties.

Another way to prioritize is to take it **one day at a time**. Breaking things down into bite-sized pieces and focusing on what must be managed immediately, rather than looking at the whole ordeal, makes cancer (like any big project) seem more manageable.

Distraction is a great tool for people confronted with a distressing situation that they cannot change. Activities that provide pleasure or an opportunity for mastery can be a major source of comfort. Some people find that working and interacting with colleagues keep their minds engaged; for others, socializing with friends and family taps into the positive feelings associated with being "normal." Even the simplest tasks and routines, such as walking the dog or completing the morning chores, can create enough divergence to allow our minds to rest from the constant stress.

Using your thoughts to **stay in the moment** and make it better can also be an effective strategy. Reminding yourself that you do have strengths and can manage, giving yourself a mental vacation by pampering yourself for a while, and using guided imagery to distract, soothe, or even bolster self-confidence are all approaches to making you feel better about yourself for a time. String a few moments together and you can give yourself a little relief from the stress.

At the extreme end of the scale in managing stress is **containment**. When Jamie was a patient, he didn't want to know about his cancer or his treatment. If doctors had information about his care or questions about how he was doing, he referred them to his wife, who could take it all in and answer. As long as he didn't have to think about the course of his cancer, he was able to manage his stress and get on with his life. While not avoiding reality, he effectively managed his problem by off-loading responsibility to a trusted soul mate.

Mind/Body Coping

Take a deep breath. Just breathe. Relax. We've all heard that advice. Turns out, it's really good guidance for dealing with stress; it brings together the mind and the body, thinking

continued

and doing. **Self-soothing** activities that focus on the five senses help us live in our bodies and enjoy a break from what's going on in our minds. Some people find pleasure in looking at a beautiful flower or listening to music that evokes a sense of calm. Smelling fresh bread, savoring a piece of chocolate, and taking a warm bath are all ways to signal to the body to let go of anxiety. While these strategies won't make the underlying issue go away, they are restorative, helping you better deal with the stress when you return to it. **Massage** is another body therapy that affects the mind. Not only does it feel good, but studies at Memorial Sloan Kettering have shown that it reduces pain, fatigue, and anxiety in cancer patients.

Prayer and **meditation** evoke a relaxation response that quiets the body, reduces stress, and promotes healing. Concentrating on the repetitive sounds of prayer focuses the mind and redefines the mind/body connection, allowing us to get a little distance from the automatic physical response to stress. Studies show they lower your heart rate, reduce blood pressure, and settle your nervous system.

Similarly, **mindfulness** is a way to bring attention to what is happening in the moment without judgment or reflection, and has been proven to shrink the amygdala and help regulate the stress response. **Yoga, progressive relaxation**, and **guided imagery** are all practices that encourage mindfulness and help turn down the level of stress hormones in the brain. Acknowledging our thoughts and releasing them is a useful way to become unstuck from difficult emotions. There are free websites and apps to help you learn and practice these techniques at home, and many cancer centers offer classes and group sessions.

If one way of coping isn't working, try another and another until you find one that works for you. With practice, you'll become more resilient, better able to handle life's stresses and with a greater capacity to recover from setbacks, face fears, and maintain hope. People who are resilient experience less stress and anxiety, so there is less wear and tear. But if your stress levels continue to climb, consider seeking professional help. Many cancer treatment programs offer psychosocial support, including one-on-one counseling, individual peer-mentoring programs, and support groups.

WHO AM I? THE MAYHEM
OF ONGOING TREATMENT

*Chaos demands to be recognized
and experienced before letting itself
be converted into a new order.*

—Hermann Hesse

As treatment wears on, many of us find ourselves struggling. The initial resolve to be strong and fight gives way to frustration and confusion as fatigue sets in and time slows to a standstill. Impatient to be well, to return to precancer life, we begin to feel hopeless. Determination gives way to depression, cognitive impairment and chaos take over, and we lose sight of who we really are. Nearly 70 percent of cancer patients report feeling stress and anxiety,[1] up to 60 percent experience fatigue or cognitive issues during and after treatment, and nearly half of all patients suffer clinically significant depression, turning into major depression for 16 percent of them.[2] This is a tough time, and few of us are prepared for these emotional complications on top of everything else we have to deal with.

"The fatigue is incredible," said Alan, sixty-five years old, in the middle of treatment for pancreatic cancer. "I lost four and a half days to fatigue so severe that I slept the entire time. I just couldn't get enough energy together to get out of bed. I'm pretty committed to my faith and synagogue, but I didn't even make it to services for the Day of Atonement, the most important day of the year. I slept practically twenty-four hours, I was so weak from the chemo."

Bill, a pianist who dedicated his life to music after retiring from software engineering, struggled with side effects from immunotherapy for Non-Hodgkin's lymphoma. "It seemed to work, but I felt as if I was losing focus; I couldn't concentrate on my music. It's hard to know if it was the disease or side effects of the treatment or just plain old age, but it was pretty unnerving. There's a family history of dementia, so I worried treatment might be hastening the inevitable."

Leslie got exasperated by the lingering cognitive effects of chemotherapy for her breast cancer. "I was used to being fairly sharp, picking up on things quickly," she said, "but that was not the case in treatment. I couldn't remember things when talking to people, had problems following conversations, and frequently asked people to repeat things. When I told my doctor I had three questions for him, but after the first one, couldn't remember the other two, he told me it was the chemo. It's so frustrating, particularly at work where I have to manage other people."

Depression

For most people, the results of treatment are cumulative—both the beneficial effects and the unfortunate repercussions. That was certainly Jillian's experience when ongoing treatment for breast cancer left her in disarray. "The very first chemo threw me into menopause overnight when I was not yet in perimeno-pause—that was the first shock," she said. "Then came the chemo brain. The keys would be in the refrigerator, or I'd have put the toast away in the cabinet—wacky stuff. And I became repetitive and unable to process thoughts as fast as I used to. I was always a little flighty, so most people didn't notice much, but I did. I felt so old."

After sixteen rounds of chemo, she finally thought the worst was behind her. Then she started taking tamoxifen. "I had always been very upbeat, but it made me suicidal," she said. "I remember thinking I could just drive into a tree or off a bridge. I knew these weren't normal thoughts, so I called my doctor, who switched my treatment to Arimidex [anas-trozole], but that is no picnic either. Now I've got chronic pain, osteoporosis, and joint pain, and I've gained twenty-five pounds. You march right through the treatment, but then there are all these other things they don't tell you about. It was overwhelming."

Carl was in the middle of interferon treatments for his mel-anoma when depression hit him. "I was a wreck," he said. "I was in the car on the way to buy a Ping-Pong table for the kids and just started sobbing. My son said, 'Daddy, it's okay.' And that just made me sob all the more. I couldn't see any hope in anything, couldn't talk to people, didn't have the energy to bother with words. I was in a hole and getting deeper, but I didn't want to quit the treatments."

Denise had neoadjuvant chemotherapy—treatment to shrink her breast cancer tumors before surgery—that left her feeling extremely anxious. "They don't really know anything about your cancer until they take it out," she said, "and waiting twenty weeks just seemed forever. At first it wasn't too bad, but the steroids made me nuts—I was bouncing off the walls. Crazy. I definitely had chemo brain, and trouble sleeping and eating. As the weeks wore on, I became a total mess—anxious, depressed, and just going through the motions of life. I didn't want my son to see me like that, so I started seeing a psychiatrist, who put me on Ativan [lorazepam] for my anxiety, and an antidepressant. I didn't want to take more drugs, but I wouldn't have managed without them."

Eileen's depression hit while she was in the hospital recovering from surgery to relieve some of the complications of mesothelioma, an incurable cancer with a limited life-expectancy after diagnosis.

> I was in the ICU [intensive care unit], in so much pain, had a rash no one could figure out, there were four drains coming out of my chest—I was miserable. Despite being a really good Catholic, I understood the benefit of doctor-assisted suicide. The next day, a priest came in wearing a beautiful white robe, with a red band around his chest. I told him I felt real despair and wanted to end it. He prayed for me and assured me my despair was not uncommon. It was so freeing to be able to confess and feel cleansed, and it really helped to know that other people suffer, too. That's what got me through as I slowly recovered and got more distracted with life.

Who Am I?

The onslaught of physical and emotional changes during this time can also challenge a patient's sense of self. As Diane said of being treated for ovarian cancer at age fifty-one, "I really questioned who this woman in the mirror was. I saw this person looking back at me, but I didn't think it was me. I was used to having energy, being competent, having strength. These things were so much a part of my identity; to not to have them was very difficult."

Patricia, dealing with breast cancer, her husband's simultaneous lung cancer, and two young children, seconded that idea. "I was someone who could work all night and be strong the next day. But the fatigue was overwhelming. When you have the sense that you're not able to rely on yourself anymore, it's disconcerting. Who are you if you don't have that?"

"Cancer challenged my feeling of worthiness," said Catherine, a psychologist diagnosed with breast cancer. "What did I do to deserve this? Mostly the answer is 'Nothing.' People who smoke every day don't get cancer, and people who never smoke do; there is no connection, but I couldn't help asking myself. Of course, the answer is, 'You don't deserve this, it just happens,' but that can be hard to remember when you are in the middle of it."

The identity issues can come in spades for someone with complex or ongoing cancer. Jeremy, the service member who retired after twenty-two years in the air force, found that out the hard way when he was being treated for pseudomyxoma peritonei, an advanced cancer that starts in the appendix and spreads throughout the abdomen.

> Mentally, I deal with it, but it sucks. I used to be able to run a mile and a half in under ten minutes,

but I'm not the physical man I once was. I am the same person, but don't get to do all that stuff I used to do. I feel seventy-five in a forty-six-year-old body. I'm not contributing to the house as I would like to, I don't behave the way my friends do (not even my unfit friends), and I can't even get a beer with them because of the medication I am on. I'm also no longer part of the working loop, so friends forget about me. I don't know who I am anymore.

For Terri, who had a family history of breast and ovarian cancer and started getting mammograms at age twenty-three, the identity issues didn't surface until she was well into breast cancer treatment.

I didn't identify with being a cancer patient. I was thirty years old, vibrant, working in the tech industry, and I didn't project that whole thing onto my life. It wasn't until my third chemo when I felt terrible that I said to myself, "No wonder I feel bad; I have cancer." But it still wasn't my identity. It was just something I was dealing with. That was surprising. I thought it would feel like it looks. Instead, it just felt like the most boring, hard marathon of my life.

But later, it created such broad identity questions for me: "Who am I, and why am I here?" "What if I die?" "And if I am going to die young, how do I look back and remember my life?" I was asking all these existential questions, but my friends and colleagues hadn't had a reason to go there yet. They hadn't experienced a struggle like cancer. I felt so alone. I didn't know how to be with the people in my life— they didn't get me.

Issues Close to Home

Physical and emotional changes also create issues with our key relationships. If you don't feel like yourself, how do you know how to interact with those you love? Claire had a tough time balancing the side effects from chemo and radiation after her double mastectomy. "The medication to prevent nausea made me constipated and my stomach was so unsettled, it made me so depressed," she said. A forty-year-old working mother with a hectic life and young kids, she found it hard to cope even with a strong support network. "How was I supposed to go back to work and continue chemo and deal with the kids and life?" But as hard as the fatigue and other physical symptoms were, it was the emotional ones that really threw her.

> I wasn't really prepared for the waves of emotions, the daily insults. My husband and I would take turns crying and being strong for each other. But there are so many lows, like realizing that I look like a ten-year-old boy but without nipples. Dealing with all these daily insults, like seeing yourself with your clothes off or worrying that others might see you differently, is exhausting. Maybe now that I look more normal, people will no longer treat me with kid gloves, but when bathing suit season comes, the kids are going to notice I don't have breasts anymore.

I don't even know how my husband feels about my body. Is he still attracted to me? My hair was always more important to me than my boobs, but a large part of my sexuality is gone, and I feel so different. We haven't had sex since my diagnosis. I feel bad for my husband—he didn't have surgery—and he must be thinking about it, but I'm sure he's hesitant to bring up the subject. I'm working toward it, but the desire hasn't been there.

Jill R. also struggled with image issues after a double mastectomy. "I never realized how distressing the disfigurement would be for me," she said. "I was not that focused on my body, but you really do feel like a freak without your breasts. I wanted to look like a normal woman, to have a sense a wholeness. I never could have imagined how a mastectomy, and the lack of hair, rob you of that feeling."

There are lots of ways that breast cancer can affect intimacy. For Noreen, who had a double mastectomy and TRAM flap reconstruction (which uses abdominal tissue to rebuild the breasts), it wasn't the loss of her breasts that was the issue. "I felt intact, no less Noreen than I was before," she said. "But the surgery brought about so many changes that having sex again with my husband took forever. My lower stomach area hurt." (She had had an incision from hip to hip, and several inches of skin and tissue rearranged for the reconstruction.) "My husband was frightened to put any weight on me, and I didn't have the strength to be on top. And then it became clear that the abdominal surgery changed the way my vagina fit. There's nothing I can do about it, but it changed me."

Intimacy can be an even bigger issue for patients who aren't in relationships. "I'm not married, but I want to have a relationship again," said Stephanie, who was disappointed with the results of her reconstruction after a double mastectomy three years earlier. "It's a huge issue. One of my implants is a little higher than the other, and the plastic surgeon said it's good enough, I said, 'Good enough for who?' People have said I'll meet someone special and it won't matter, but I'm not sure I want to be with someone for whom it won't matter."

While breast cancer creates some obvious ramifications for sexual intimacy, patients with other types of cancers suffer too. As Nancy I. put it, "Forget trying to have a sex life after you have your ovaries removed! It's too painful. I tease my husband all the time: 'Do you have someone on the side?'"

SCIENCE SIDEBAR: WHEN DISEASE AND TREATMENT TAKE YOUR LIFE AWAY

Many of us going through cancer treatment are so thankful to be alive, we don't think we have a right to expect a sex life too, but sex is a part of living. It feels good, contributes to a sense of vitality, releases hormones that create a warm glow long after the sex is over, and helps us maintain intimacy with our partners. But sex and cancer don't always play together nicely. Research shows that 30 to 100 percent of cancer patients have some type of sexual difficulty.[3] And with good reason. As if the psychological stress and loss of sense of self that come with being deep into cancer treatment weren't enough, there are some very real physical changes that interfere with sexuality for nearly all cancer patients, starting with fatigue.

When you are saving every ounce of energy to get through the day, it can be hard to find the personal resources to initiate or respond to sexual activity. But it's not just that we are tired. Fatigue and its corollary, inflammation, make it hard to feel sexy. As we saw in chapter 3, inflammation is caused by pro-inflammatory cytokines, chemical messengers that tell the brain how to deal with threats and encourage "sickness behavior." And while that sickness behavior may drive us back to bed, it's not with any pleasurable intent in mind.

It's not just that sickness behavior makes us feel tired. Inflammation reduces the sex drive. In one study, 65 percent of patients receiving treatment with interferon, a naturally occurring pro-inflammatory cytokine that is used to stimulate the immune system in treating cancer and other diseases, reported a decline in libido, correlating with a marked decline in sex hormones during treatment.[4] A second study shows that infusion with interleukin, another pro-inflammatory cytokine, leads to decreases in testosterone,[5] and loss of libido is a common symptom for those with chronic inflammation, such as rheumatoid arthritis sufferers and tuberculosis patients.[6] So clearly anyone being treated with cytokine therapy is likely to feel the effects, but we know that surgery, radiation, and medical oncology treatments all lead to increases in cytokine activity, so hormonal changes are likely a factor for many of us.

Unfortunately, the obstacles to a healthy sex life during cancer treatment don't stop there. Any surgery on the neck, abdomen, or pelvis, especially if it results in temporary drains or permanent ostomies, has the ability to disrupt intimacy. Incisional pain and tenderness can make physical contact difficult. Breathing may be challenging, and muscles may not work the way they did before the operation. Surgery for breast, testicular, prostate, gynecologic, and colorectal cancers can damage nerves, creating physical sensitivities at our most intimate sites, or even jeopardizing the control of blood flow necessary for erection or vaginal lubrication.[7] Nearly 60 percent of women with breast cancer say pain and discomfort were driving factors in their reduced sexual activity after cancer.[8] And for some women, breast reconstruction after treatment can add months of tenderness and pain. A third of women have reconstruction complications that delay recovery.[9]

Women who have hysterectomies may end up with

continued

anatomical changes that affect their sex lives for the long-term, and if their ovaries are removed, they may have significant hormonal changes even if they were already in menopause. Meanwhile, impotence and incontinence are not uncommon for men undergoing prostate surgery and may be slow to resolve.[10] And brain cancer surgery carries a unique risk: damaging the control center for sexual activity and pleasure. While research in this area is still limited, sexual dysfunction is a complication for some brain cancer patients, especially those undergoing surgery for tumors in the temporal lobe.[11]

Radiation also can take a toll, increasing sensitivity or even resulting in burning, peeling, thickening, and scarring of the skin. Long after the skin has healed, its texture and sensitivity may be different; touch that was once pleasurable may now be painful, or without sensation. While that's bad enough when it's on the outside (on the breasts or abdomen), it's even worse when it's on the inside (in the vagina) and can lead to narrowing that makes intercourse virtually impossible, at least for a time. In addition to causing skin changes, pelvic radiation can damage nerves, resulting in neuropathy or incontinence. For some folks, this disruption is short-lived, while for others, normal sensation never returns.

And then there's chemotherapy. In addition to the general fatigue, weakness, and anemia that many chemo agents create, some affect blood flow, which can make it difficult for people to feel aroused. Many of these agents reduce libido, and some, especially taxanes and platinum drugs, lead to skin sensitivities, nerve damage, and inflammation that can affect the sex organs.[12]

How about hormone therapy? Androgen-deprivation therapy for prostate cancer and hormone suppression for estrogen-positive cancers or as a result of ovary-removal surgery significantly reduce libido, increase anxiety and emotional lability, and can lead to depression—not exactly making us feel sexy.[13] And then there are the physical symptoms, such as vaginal dryness, pelvic pain, erectile dysfunction, penile shortening, and pain with intercourse. In addition to the direct hit these hormone-deprivation drugs cause, they also can interfere with recovery. Estrogen plays a role in reducing inflammation, so without its benefit, the bodies of men and women on hormone-suppression drugs have a harder time regaining cytokine balance.[14] Inflammation hangs around longer, libido stays suppressed longer, and the fatigue and sickness behavior continue to plague us.

Many patients, as part of their chemo- or immune-therapy treatments, take steroids to suppress an immune reaction to the treatments, increase their effectiveness, and decrease inflammation. These, too, can interfere with sex; increased levels of cortisol and its synthetic alternatives (such as prednisone and dexamethasone) suppress testosterone, mess with the HPA axis (see the Science Sidebar in chapter 1), and generally decrease libido.

While many of these problems resolve as treatment ends and patients recover, some linger for months or even years after the treatment is finished. Drains come out, scars fade, hormones stabilize, damaged nerves quiet down, and our

continued

bodies and minds adjust to the new realities of life, but maybe the stoma is permanent, or the hormone deprivation therapy is long-term, or the skin damage unyielding. Sometimes we need medical interventions. Topical lidocaine for ongoing nerve pain, lubricants and vaginal dilators for stenosis, hormone supplementation to address imbalances, Viagra for erectile dysfunction—oncologists know which symptoms are related to the disease or treatment, what has worked for other patients with similar issues, and what is most likely to work for you. But more likely than not, it's up to you to ask about it. Fewer than 14 percent of patients with sexual difficulties report that their medical teams initiated a conversation about sex.[15] So if your sex life has been affected by cancer and its treatment, talk to your medical team. Sexual intimacy is a normal part of a healthy life, and your doctor can help, but only if she knows there is a problem. Make a list of your concerns, and don't be embarrassed to discuss them at your next visit. You, and your partner, will be glad you did.

In addition to disrupting physical intimacy, cancer can create an experiential distance that can lead to gaps in emotional intimacy. "I destroyed my marriage with my first cancer," said Steve, undergoing treatment for colon cancer after having survived testicular cancer more than twenty-five years earlier. "I pushed my wife away—didn't want to accept anyone's support. I felt like I was the only one going through this, that no one knew how I felt, and that made a wall between us."

Of course, patients are not the only ones struggling with their emotions during cancer. Often, intimate loved ones are just as challenged by the whole ordeal. Cass, who was sixty-one when she had breast cancer, found that the experience disrupted her marriage as well. "My husband was not really available to me when I was sick," she said. "He's been very dependent on me because he has heart disease and was terrified. He thought I was going to leave him, so he withdrew and was not at all supportive."

Blair, diagnosed with chronic lymphocytic leukemia at age forty-three, had a similar experience. "My husband was very scared with my diagnosis," she said. "He freaked out. He was there, physically, and doing things to take care of the kids and the house, but I didn't feel supported. His tolerance for me being sick got lower and lower as the weeks went by. I tried not to complain, but the tension between us kept growing. At one point, he got mad at me and said, 'What the fuck, why can't you just get better?' It was like he had a certain amount of empathy, and after he had used that up, there was nothing left."

While the mayhem of ongoing treatment creates special challenges for couples, it's a difficult time for many patients, worn down by treatment and the struggles of the prior months. For many, the ordeal may soon be over, but sometimes, anxiety and continued physical and emotional turmoil make recovery feel like an unattainable goal.

SIDEBAR: Q AND A
ON INTIMACY ISSUES

Psychotherapists support patients through all types of emotional issues, including the challenges that arise with cancer. Some patients find psychosocial support as an integral part of their treatment programs at cancer centers and hospitals; others seek support through community resources and independent professionals. **Sara R. Pasternak, PhD**, is an **independent clinical psychologist** whose early research in coping with pain and cancer at Memorial Sloan Kettering Cancer Center (MSKCC) led to her specialty in treating patients with medical illnesses. **A clinical advisor to Mount Sinai Hospital's Woman to Woman peer-mentoring program for gynecologic cancer patients and a former consulting psychologist at MSKCC,** she helps patients with a variety of emotional needs, including anxiety, depression, PTSD, and dealing with relationships and intimacy issues, while continuing to focus on patients coping with cancer.

Why is intimacy a particular challenge for cancer patients?

Intimacy is hard for everyone. As a society, we are not very good at talking about it—particularly sexual intimacy. And even in the closest relationships, there is a natural gap between people, so maintaining the relationship requires constant attention. Someone dealing with cancer may not have the time or energy to devote to maintaining closeness—when you are in crisis, naturally everything else gets pushed aside. Plus, there is the stress of the diagnosis itself, which interferes with normal functioning. You can't help but be distracted and wrapped up in your own fears when dealing with an existential threat, so it's easy to get a little out of synch. You may not even realize that you are excluding your partner from your fears or from bits of information you are learning, which contributes to a growing gap between you. When you add to that the physical and emotional issues that result from the disease and its treatment, it is not surprising that intimacy is a particular challenge.

When patients express concerns about intimacy, what are some of the specific emotional issues that typically come up?

In addition to the growing sense of estrangement between a couple going through cancer together, body image, fear, and mismatched libido are the issues that most frequently complicate intimacy. You may not feel the same about your body, or even feel ashamed by the changes the disease and its treatment caused. This can lead to worries that your partner won't find you attractive anymore, or even reduce your own desire for sex. Or maybe you don't even know that you are ready to have sex again. Alternatively, you may still feel attractive and have a healthy drive but may wonder if your partner still finds you so. Sometimes you feel rejected because your partner is avoiding sex out of respect for you, afraid that suggesting sex would be selfish. "How can I be

continued

thinking about sex when she is facing so many challenges?" Fear that sex will be painful—for you or your partner—is also a common issue, as well as worries about performing as expected. All of these concerns are indicative of a gap that can easily grow during a time of stress, whether related to an illness or some other disruption, like having children. It's natural that intimacy changes, and it's natural that it can come back, but it doesn't just happen spontaneously. You have to put some effort into it—adjusting to change takes time.

After a break in sexual activity for surgery and treatment, what can patients do to signal their readiness and initiate intimacy with their partners?

Reestablishing intimacy takes two things—prioritizing the couple again, and being able to communicate, verbally and nonverbally. When people are first attracted to one another, they make time to get to know each other—to establish a bond and become a couple. It can be helpful to remember what it was like when you first met, what first attracted you to each other, and how much effort you put into thinking about each other. If you can remember those feelings, there is a good chance you can recreate them.

Prioritizing time for each other again can be hard with the additional burdens of care or the catching up after all that. Saying something as simple as "I want to spend time together" elevates the needs of the couple and sends a signal—not that we are going to jump into bed together, but rather a signal that you want to start focusing on being a couple again. Maybe you go for a walk and hold hands. Maybe you have a lazy meal and really look at one another again. Or maybe you cuddle on the couch while watching TV together. Just creating a special time that a couple can count on sharing, as one might share a bedtime ritual with a child, lays the groundwork for reestablishing intimacy. Even fifteen minutes with no talk about medical or household things can make a difference. But it takes time, and you have to do it again and again.

I also encourage couples to go out. When you first met each other, you were on neutral territory, not in the home, which can be laden with responsibilities and memories, particularly post-care. Everyone can move through those memories with time, but if you're trying to get things revitalized, it helps to break the routine, to find the spontaneity and court your partner again.

Sometimes that's enough to kick-start sexual intimacy because both of you are ready and wondering about the other. But if it's not happening naturally, the next step is to communicate, and how you do that depends on how you are as a couple. Some couples are playful, and saying, "I'm ready," in an outrageous and funny way may be all it takes. Other couples are more shy with each other and would find that approach insulting or off-putting. Sometimes, saying, "What aren't we talking about?" may bring the conversation around to sex without having to bluntly raise it. It really depends on the couple, but whatever is said, it's best to begin with something positive or neutral. A negative statement rarely gets you anywhere, and the worst thing to do is

continued

to start with an accusation. Saying something like "I don't think you like me anymore" or "You don't find me attractive anymore" puts your partner in a defensive mode and doesn't acknowledge any of your own contributions to the emotional distance. Have you been sharing as much as you used to? Are you the same as you were before the diagnosis? It also negates any fears or concerns that your partner may be feeling, including "I'm so afraid for you and here I am doing everything I can to be supportive and don't you see that?"

When you resume having sex, you may need to talk about yourself, what feels good and what doesn't, what exactly you want your partner to do, just as you may have guided your partner the first time you had sex. Give it time. It won't happen overnight, but if you both are willing to make the effort and anticipate a few ups and downs, you can rekindle the intimacy.

What about when patients don't have a steady partner? When and how should they bring up cancer when dating and trying to establish new partnerships?

If a couple is dating but not yet in a committed relationship, it can be very hard to navigate a cancer diagnosis. Often, they don't yet have enough experience or "glue" as a couple to know how to manage, and it becomes less about intimacy and more about vulnerability—who feels most vulnerable and least able to accommodate the change. In some forming couples, the patient may feel bad about being a burden, or conversely, may need more support and reassurance than the partner is able to give. At the same time, the partner can become selfless, putting the patient first without recognizing the personal sacrifice and later not knowing how to cope with that, or may end the relationship, feeling overwhelmed by the needs of a new partner. Finding the balance so you both feel you chose to support each other through the crisis will take open communication and trust, and can lay the groundwork for a powerful long-term relationship.

For people who are just dating, knowing when to tell someone about your cancer can be tricky. Too soon, and you scare off a potential partner before a relationship has a chance to blossom. Too late, and you come across as secretive at a time when you are trying to build trust. It's best to raise the subject when the relationship starts to get serious, or when you are ready for sexual intimacy. Your partner will likely respond to how you present the information as much as to the news itself, so think about what you want to convey and how that might be perceived. It can be helpful to practice in advance, so you know what you want to say and can get comfortable saying it. It's also important to recognize that how you feel about it and what you want to say are likely to change over time. The physical and emotional scars fade over time, and the urgency about addressing them can also melt away.

When body-image issues arise, how do you coach people and their partners to get beyond them?

When a patient goes through cancer, there can be a lot of physical changes, not all of which are anticipated. Maybe you knew you would have a scar, or maybe you anticipated

continued

hair loss from chemo, but you might not anticipate weight loss or even weight gain. You might be surprised by how the fatigue makes you look older, or how the changes in your skin from chemo or radiation make you feel less like yourself. Try to take it slowly. It may take a while for your body to get back to normal and for you to get comfortable with your new normal. These changes may affect how you think about yourself, which affects your emotions and your self-image.

Most of us focus on our weak points and tend to be far more critical of ourselves than others are of us. If you're having trouble adjusting to how you look now, you might want to start by focusing on your best features. Maybe you always liked your strong jawline, or the soft skin on the inside of your arms. Those probably haven't changed, and by finding ways to emphasize the features you like best, you may feel better about yourself. Look at yourself fully clothed in the mirror. Can you see the features you always used to like about yourself? What are the features that a total stranger would notice about you? What would a stranger say to compliment you? When you can see your good points fully clothed, the next step is to translate that into feeling good about yourself while semiclothed and then naked. Can you disguise the things you don't like about yourself? Can you wear a teddy to hide your ostomy bag? Would a different type of underwear hide your weight loss? Get creative and see if you can give yourself a compliment or two.

When you are comfortable with the disguises, begin to look at yourself in the nude. Is that scar really as bad as you think? Would someone who loves you see you or see the scar? Can you remember the compliments you gave yourself when you were fully clothed? Once you have reached a point where you can accept these changes, then explain to your partner how you have adjusted to them. Sometimes it is nonverbal—take your partner's finger and trace your scars to show that you are not uncomfortable with them.

Most body changes come on gradually, giving us plenty of time to adjust. We don't see the effects of aging on a daily basis or notice when our hair falls out, but when you have cancer, changes can happen quickly, and it takes time to get comfortable with them. Be kind to yourself and take it slowly. Exercise can help you remember what your body is for, and help you feel pleasure in using it, even if you are not yet finding pleasure in looking at it.

What can patients do when they are no longer aroused by the behaviors and sexual patterns that always used to work?

When a patient's physical sensations have changed, it can be hard to communicate that something that always worked before doesn't anymore. But that communication is essential. It may be a guiding hand or it may be a direct statement; that's up to you and what feels comfortable. Sometimes saying something in a matter-of-fact way at the least-intimate moment and then walking away can diffuse the tension of it, such as, "I was talking to my doctor and this is what he said, and we will figure this out together." It's information, and there is no need to respond to it at that moment, but now it

continued

is out there. Or you can say, "This is what's different for me now, and I don't know what the answer is, but we can have some fun figuring this out together." Or even, "I don't know what's going to work and I wonder about it." It's an open invitation for help without any judgment or demand.

Sex may not be great to start with, but don't be discouraged. Keep trying. It's not anyone's fault and there is no shame. It's just different. And it may continue to change. For some couples, sex becomes better than before cancer because they actually start talking about their fantasies and experimenting in ways they hadn't. Try candles, erotic movies, sex toys. Anything is possible. There are lots of different ways to have pleasure, and there are ways to find physical satisfaction in being close. But if it is uncomfortable, stop. Don't perpetuate something that hurts and try not to let your frustration affect an intimate moment. Instead, pleasure each other in a different way, or take a break and just cuddle. Sex shouldn't be something that adds to your list of worries.

When should patients seek the advice of a mental health professional to support them with intimacy issues?

In general, if something is interfering with your happiness and satisfaction in life, then you need to look at it, particularly if it is getting in the way of your self-esteem. If you are working through it and feel you are making progress, then keep at it, but if you seem stuck as a couple, it's best to ask for help. Sometimes the stress around intimacy issues can be disguised as fighting about who is going to take out the garbage. You may not be addressing the underlying tension head-on, but it's there and interfering with life. That's when you need to be in a room together and talk through the challenges you are experiencing, and having a third person might help facilitate that conversation.

It is also helpful to seek support when there is shame or feelings of guilt and responsibility associated with getting cancer. If you feel guilty, it can be very hard to allow intimacy back in your life. I try to break down those feelings to understand the source. Sometimes, guilt is disguised as wanting more control or thinking you had more control to start with. "If only I had stopped smoking sooner, or eaten more fish, I could have prevented my cancer." Hanging on to this sense of guilt helps you avoid an understanding of the randomness of cancer that makes people feel so vulnerable. If you think you had some control and still you got cancer, you blew it, so you feel guilty. But it's overwhelming to realize that you have no control—that you have to confront the existential question of the unpredictability of life. Guilt is an acceptable way of getting encouragement, but its damage to feelings of self-worth are an added challenge to intimacy.

For more information and support in dealing with issues of sexual intimacy, go to the American Cancer Society's Treatment and Support section at https://www.cancer.org/treatment/treatments-and-side-effects/physical-side-effects/fertility-and-sexual-side-effects.html.

ADVICE FROM THOSE WHO LEARNED IT THE HARD WAY

Getting through treatment is hard—it's physically and emotionally draining. In fact, the word "patient" comes from the Latin word for suffering. After months of distress, it's no wonder we are *impatient*, or anxious to be done. While "keep a stiff upper lip" and "all in good time" may be applicable advice, platitudes sound hollow in the midst of our misery. But there are some things we can do to help get through this phase of the ordeal.

Many patients have found they were self-critical or disappointed in their reserves as treatment wore on, and advise others to be more tolerant. As Catherine said, "Be gentle, loving, and patient with yourself. It's an incredibly intense time. Even when you feel crazy and like you are going to lose it, remember you're not going to feel like that forever. Just allow yourself to feel the anger and everything else that passes over you." Shilpi echoed that advice. "You have to take the long view on it because the day-to-day can get very dreary. It's overwhelming—and then you are on the other side and getting better." Or, as Denise put it, "Remember how strong you are. As sucky as it is, you'll be okay."

It can be hard to find the strength to go through one more day when you also are concerned with how others may be perceiving you and your cancer struggle. But Leslie said, reminding us of our priorities, "Don't worry about other people. Focus on you, and just know that what you are feeling isn't unusual or wrong."

Unfortunately, as Steve pointed out, "People are very uncomfortable around cancer. We are taught as little kids that it's a deadly disease and people die from it. So I joke with my friends about it and give them license to do the same. I don't want them treating me any differently. I know I need them in my life and will get more support from them if my cancer is just part of our normal relationship."

Joking, teasing, and finding some way to laugh or smile can make a difference. "Attitude is everything—so much a part of how you handle things and how you heal," said Jillian. "You've got two choices: to be happy or to be depressed. It can be hard for some folks, but finding something to be joyful about made it more tolerable. People would ask, 'Why are you so fucking happy?' I was joyful I had such amazing support, joyful that this wasn't a permanent state, even if it seemed to last forever."

As Terri said, "When you light up, it brings joy. Think about what lights you up and trust that." For Eileen, it was her religion that helped her smile and transcend the wretchedness of ongoing treatment. "Having faith in something that goes beyond the material can be a big source of strength. I don't know how I would have gotten through without it." Even finding absurdities to chuckle about can bring you strength. As Alan said, "I grew up in a dysfunctional household. Now I'm thankful that I learned how to live with chaos and denial. Who would have thought that would have been a wonderful inheritance?"

Perhaps the most important advice, however, is to communicate, to share, to let people know how you feel. As Carl said, "Try not to be isolated; talk to your loved ones about what you are going through. How are they supposed to understand if you don't?" Elyse said, "People who love you want to help, if you let them. It can be hard to ask for help, but allow yourself to accept the need for support."

Even if you don't have loved ones around you who are supportive, you can find people who understand what you are going through. Most hospitals and cancer centers have support groups, and many have peer-to-peer mentoring programs. In addition, Cancer Support Community, (https://www.cancersupportcommunity.org), Imerman Angels (https://imermanangels.org), and Cancer Hope Network (https://www.cancerhopenetwork.org) will find a peer mentor who has been through your cancer and treatment and who will connect with you in person, on the phone, or through email. Sometimes just knowing that you are not alone in your cancer or your emotions can make all the difference.

SCANXIETY: TESTING AND MONITORING DURING AND AFTER TREATMENT

*"All anxiety is because of a desire
for harmony. Seek disharmony,
then you will gain peace."*

—*Rumi*

Nobody likes getting medical tests. Whether from a needle stick for a simple blood test, a breast-smashing mammogram, a claustrophobia-inducing MRI or CT scan, or a painfully invasive cystoscopy, there is some measure of physical discomfort associated with just about every form of medical testing. But for most patients, it's not the physical discomfort that brings anxiety. It is the heightened sense of uncertainty as we are reminded, yet again, that we had cancer, that it may not be gone, that it may come back. Studies report that fear of recurrence is nearly universal,[1] although the percentage of patients for whom this anxiety reaches "clinically significant" levels is much smaller, with estimates ranging from 30 to 40 percent.[2] As Monica said, "Fifty percent of people with my cancer recur. I'm now at the point where I can either let myself relax and believe that I will have a long life, or remind myself that I have cancer and that might not happen. I don't want to live in fear, but don't want to live my life foolishly either."

That uncertainty about the future can be unsettling. Deborah wants to remain optimistic, but sometimes it can be challenging. "My ob-gyn said I was cured," she said. "But we don't really know. You never know which side of the odds you're on and if it's coming back." Or, as Alan said, "I think I'm done, and my pattern of denial helps keep the fear away, but in the back of my mind, I worry. Pancreatic cancer can be a very fast killer, and that fear is still there. I suspect it is at the root of my irritability even though it is not in my conscious mind 24/7."

And that presence in the back of the mind can lead cancer survivors to be hypochondriacs. Three years after her treatment ended, Charlotte said, "I still get a little freaked out by random symptoms. The doctor told me to be aware of changes in my breasts, in my bones, in my liver. So if I get an unexplainable twinge, I assume it's cancer coming back. When my back hurt, I went to the ER [emergency room] and was assured it wasn't cancer. I may be a little paranoid about it, but I'd rather be safe."

Anticipating Disaster

As patients, we are hypervigilant after the initial diagnosis and treatment, following a prescribed regimen of doctors' visits and tests with a frequency declining from weekly or monthly to annual checkups. Many of us are told that the risk of recurrence or treatment failure is greatest in the beginning—that if we can make it to the magical five-year mark, we can consider ourselves cured. So we come to anticipate these checkups with true ambivalence; we want the reassurance of having passed another milestone but fear what the tests and examinations may show. Most patients are able to put this fear aside and move on with life between medical appointments, but doctors' visits, blood tests, and scans heighten the fear. As many as 83 percent of patients experience scan-associated distress,[3] triggered by concerns about the unknown and the uncontrollable nature of what the results portend.[4] The degree of anxiety is often tied to the severity of the disease, likelihood of recurrence, and how long it's been since diagnosis, but it is rare that we get by without some angst.

Part of the anxiety comes from having learned that feeling well is not an indication that we are well—we know cancer can grow without generating any symptoms. As Elyse put it, "You don't trust your body anymore, or its healing capacity. I have the ability to spend 99 percent of two months not thinking about it, but then the sense of vulnerability comes back." Without being able to trust our own instincts, we come to rely on testing, yet many of the tests are inconclusive, leaving us dangling while we await repeated or additional testing.

"The hardest part of the whole thing was getting those tests," said Mary K., a survivor of ovarian cancer, for which a blood test looking at a specific cancer antigen is a primary indicator of the disease and its response to treatment. "After the test, when I knew the results would be back, I would pour myself a scotch, take a couple of sips, log in to the hospital website, and click on the results. If the statistic was on a downward trend (a positive sign), I would feel great for the next three months until I had to get another test, but if the trend was up, I would be a wreck, even though I knew that a repeat might show a different answer. I became obsessed with the blood test results and plotted them logarithmically for five years, and it's not even a very good indicator of the presence of cancer."

For Stephanie, the worry about cancer coming back was overwhelming. "Every three months when I would go for a checkup, I would shake. The x-rays, chest MRIs, DEXA [dual-energy x-ray absorptiometry] scans, and the blood work—it all scared me. I am sure I would be fine if the cancer came back—I would step up and deal with it—but I worry about it every time I go for testing."

As Nickie said after pancreatic cancer and multiple myeloma, "It's the not knowing, thinking that it's getting worse, wondering what's next. Mostly I don't worry about it coming back, but I do worry when it's time for tests. And when they give me the all-clear, I release that worry."

Faded Fears and Lasting Anxiety

For many patients, the passage of time is a big help. As Amy said of Eliot's metastatic melanoma, "In the beginning, we were going to the hospital so frequently getting scans that if he got a headache, it panicked me. But now, I have to remind myself that he had cancer. It just doesn't seem as real or as urgent."

Bob, three years out from his bladder cancer diagnosis, agrees. "With cancer, you don't know what's next. In the beginning, you get tested so frequently and hope you hear good news. Sometimes you even have to chase the doctors for results, so it's natural to get a little anxious around test time. Now it's still a big unknown, but doesn't feel quite as scary. I would be surprised if they found something."

For years after her ovarian cancer diagnosis, Nancy H. went for tests every three months, unwilling to relax in her vigilance about recurrence. Only recently, in conversation with a friend, did she recognize that it wasn't a driving force anymore. "She asked if I was worried all the time, and I said no, it'd been fourteen years, plus I get a cancer antigen test...and then I realized, I didn't remember when I had last had the test! It had finally stopped being top of mind. But, I did call the doctor right away to arrange to get another one!"

For others, the apprehension lingers. Brian, who had bladder cancer fifteen years ago, still gets anxious about the most basic test—the presence of blood in his urine. "I don't pee without looking," he said, "so there is still some residual anxiety."

Larry, who lost his first wife to breast cancer, agrees that testing is a high-anxiety time. "She was two weeks shy of the fifth anniversary of her diagnosis when they found another tumor, so I know there is no magic window. A lot can happen in six months. My blood pressure is off the wall when I go for my bladder cancer checkups. The anticipation, not the reality, is what is bad."

Patricia, whose breast cancer was diagnosed the same day as her husband's lung cancer, has seen anxiety levels fluctuate with changing news. "I don't really worry about my cancer coming back, but I get very anxious about his scans. We assumed everything was going to be fine, but after one bad scan, we know that isn't necessarily the case. So now I have some anxiety about what else they might find."

And when complications arise, so does anxiety. Cass had multiple setbacks with reconstruction for breast cancer. "Each setback would cause more distress. 'Why am I still having trouble?' I think I had expected that it would be easy and that I would be done, but it seems it is never truly done. Something always seems to crop up."

Sometimes, all the vigilance can lead to problems of its own. As Ellen, a breast cancer survivor, said, "When they say they are going to watch you like a hawk, there will be false alarms. I had seven months of false alarms, including when I found a new lump in my breast. It turns out to have been an oil cyst, which can form as a result of damage from a biopsy or chemo or radiation. Once we were sure it was nothing, the doctor told me to stop checking all the time and just have faith that they were watching me closely and nothing was going to happen without them knowing about it. But it's hard to stop worrying and checking."

Catherine had a similar experience. Eighteen months after her breast cancer surgery, she felt a warm spot in her armpit and was worried about a recurrence. Waiting for her positron-emission tomography (PET)/CT scan, she felt herself begin to panic. "'What if it's back? What if I die?' But I came to a place of peace with it, not wanting to die, but accepting it. Then this guy comes out saying he was 'looking for the patient who has cancer' and I said, 'I don't have cancer, I *had* cancer.' And sure enough, it was just an enlarged lymph gland."

For some patients, making peace with ambiguity seems to help. As Diane said of her tests for endometrial cancer,

"There is no certainty in any of it. The only sure thing is when someone tells you, 'You have a recurrence and we're treating you again.' You have to embrace the uncertainty because it is preferable to having cancer again!" Jane M., who has been battling one cancer or another for several years, agrees. "I got a clean scan this time," she said. "But will I get a clean scan next time? No clue. And even PET scans are nonconclusive. There are things that could be read differently by two different doctors. So you move into an uncertain realm. And when you deal with uncertainty on a regular basis, you stop fighting it."

SCIENCE SIDEBAR: REPEAT EXPOSURE AND ANXIETY

Traumatic experiences can lead to stress and anxiety, manifested in the form of intrusive thoughts or reflexive reactions or avoidance. The military has known that for decades, although the term for it has evolved with greater understanding—from "shell shock" to "combat fatigue" to modern-day PTSD. More recently, the medical community has come to recognize the trauma-inducing nature of a life-threatening diagnosis and its potential to produce stress and anxiety, establishing specific PTSD diagnosis criteria that include being told you have a life-threatening disease.[5] Just as traumatic experiences in a war zone can lead to PTSD for a soldier, so too can the diagnosis of cancer for any of us. And while sudden loud noises are a common trigger for war-induced trauma, a medical test or scan is all that is needed to remind us of the existential crisis initiated by a diagnosis of cancer.

Only 7 to 14 percent of us will develop full-blown, cancer-induced PTSD, but as many as 60 percent of us view the diagnosis and treatment of cancer as traumatic.[6] How strong a reaction we have seems to be driven by who we are at the time of the diagnosis—our genetics, brain chemistry, prior life stressors, coping styles, age, and life experience—as well as by the nature of the diagnosis: the severity of the disease, the invasiveness of treatment, and how well we are doing physically.

But other factors related to treatment can contribute to anxiety as well, including poor communication with our doctors, fear of needles, pain, medications, hormonal imbalances, shortness of breath, and even vitamin deficiencies.[7] Women are more likely to experience anxiety than men, as are those with a prior history of distress, and some cancers are more distressing than others. (Head and neck cancers, perhaps due to their disfiguring effects, are more likely to generate distress than is colon cancer.)[8] Another factor that seems to contribute to the degree of distress we feel is our ability to tolerate uncertainty. It's not just uncertainty about our own health status that's nerve-racking; it's uncertainty about how our health will affect those we love. Those of us who are uncomfortable with uncertainty tend to view it as threatening, which perpetuates anxiety. This is particularly challenging for men with diagnoses of prostate cancer, for whom the treatment may be "active surveillance,"[9] but it affects all of us being monitored during and after treatment. We can spend weeks not thinking about having cancer, but the test or scan reminds us, and leaves us with lingering uncertainty while we await results.

Although not a lot of research has been done to understand the physiology behind cancer-induced PTSD, it appears that reported levels of distress correlate with the levels of activity in brain regions involved in the stress response, especially the hypothalamus, suggesting there is a physiological response driving the anxiety.[10] Additional work has shown that the HPA axis (see the Science Sidebar in chapter 1) is out of balance in breast cancer patients reporting PTSD, resulting in lower than normal levels of cortisol and higher levels of norepinephrine.[11]

continued

Scientists have also begun to identify the specific variations in cytokine genes that lead to higher levels of anxiety among cancer patients.[12] Perhaps someday, as they sequence genes to better tailor treatment, they will also screen for the likelihood of anxiety and help us anticipate and respond to it.

Social support seems to mitigate stress. Even if you have the cytokine genes that predispose you to anxiety, the presence of a loving family caregiver can help reduce the likelihood of anxiety.[13] Unfortunately, a major source of support, the professional care team, isn't always with us. For many patients, anxiety increases when they transition away from regular contact with doctors, nurses, and chemo-suite friends after treatment. They no longer have the reassurance that a new occurrence will immediately be detected, or such easy access to support to ask about the latest unexplained twinge.

Recent research is beginning to show the benefits of mind/body interventions in addition to social support in reducing anxiety about cancer recurrence. By teaching us how to let go of intrusive thoughts and think more flexibly about the future, mindfulness meditation and cognitive behavioral therapy (CBT) can help us change our normal thought patterns and gain a bit more comfort with the uncertainty of being a cancer patient or survivor.[14] Research shows that behaviors such as meditation, yoga, repetitive prayer, and other practices that elicit the relaxation response—the biological opposite of the fight-or-flight response—create biochemical changes in the brain that promote well-being, and even change the way thousands of genes are expressed as our cells reproduce. While long-term practitioners are likely to sustain a greater and more long-lasting benefit, even one fifteen-minute session of meditation can change gene-directed immune and stress response.[15]

So when scanxiety strikes, take a deep breath. Find a yoga, tai chi, or qigong class at the local Y, inquire at your hospital about CBT, find a meditation app for your phone, go to religious services, or get a massage. Sometimes the hardest part is making the time to do it, but the payoff in a little less stress, and maybe even a better night's sleep, will soon be obvious.

ADVICE FROM THOSE WHO LEARNED IT THE HARD WAY

Finding some way to get through the repeated anxiety of testing can challenge your emotional strength and creativity. Just when you are ready to be done with it all, you are reminded again of the potential for an existential crisis. But there are some approaches that are known to help.

Many patients find that they need to psych themselves up for their tests and put on a brave front. They find that false bravado becomes real bravado when practiced with conviction. Mark suggested that the best way to deal with pretest anxiety was to be tough. "Once you get cancer, you learn that you can't wuss out," he said. "For me, it was like when I went to jail. You can't go in there scared, even if you are. It's the same thing with scans. Try not to think about it until the day before. Then it owns you," he said. "So you have to be a badass." Aparna agreed. She recommended harnessing your emotions, although she found it difficult. "Write down your fears. Keep a diary and write about what worries you. It helps to release them if you write them down."

Others recommend a more active approach to managing fear. Cass suggests, "Turn anxiety into action by doing something to help yourself, learn more, exercise more, do more of whatever helps you feel good." Carl agreed that exercise was key. "Waiting for results is like awaiting your fate—it's hard to just sit there. I would get on my bike and ride so I would be away and busy, and then exhausted and relaxed, instead of hanging by the phone."

Leslie endorsed burying yourself in the routine of work.

"Having the steady demands of a job keeps you sane, so try to carry on as normally as possible. It fills your mind and your time."

Absorbing your mind in something fun can also divert it from stress. Anne suggested finding joy. "Do things you enjoy, that make you happy. It's a great distraction from fear," she said. For Catherine, that meant turning up the heat. "Turn your anxiety into passion. You can get a great personal boost from some really great sex, and it takes the edge off the fear." Catherine also recommended exploring integrative-medicine techniques. "Guided imagery can really help, and qigong. They give you other ways of processing the fear."

Others find the calm they need in some type of mind/body practice. Meditation was the source of strength and calm for Urvi when she was most anxious. "You have to live with the doubts and learn to let go of the anxiety," she said. "I meditated every day and that helped a lot. You have to just forget the unpleasant things in life." Sue M. said, "It doesn't have to be a formal meditation; even just being mindful can help. Recognizing that there are things you can control and things you can't, and practicing letting go of the ones you can't." Jennifer suggested the benefits of prayer. "Cancer and chemo and the testing that comes along with it are hard, nothing but pure heartache, and you can't do it alone," she said. "The most heartbreaking thing is to do it alone, but with support and prayer, it makes it a whole lot better."

Getting professional support is also helpful. As Loretta said, "If anxiety from the uncertainty of cancer is making you crazy, get some professional help. It can make a huge difference. Even though my girlfriends were all rooting for me, I found myself telling them it was going to be fine. But inside

I wasn't fine. It really helps to have someone say that fear and anxiety are normal for a life-threatening experience, regardless of the physical results."

Many hospitals and cancer centers offer counseling as part of their comprehensive care. Even if you have friends and family with whom you share your feelings, if fear and anxiety are getting in the way of you functioning, sleeping, and getting on with life, speak to your doctor about getting help.

SIDEBAR: Q AND A ON INTEGRATIVE MEDICINE

Ting Bao, MD, director of integrative breast oncology and integrative medicine specialist at Memorial Sloan Kettering Cancer Center, is focused on integrating the traditional medicine of her homeland, China, with Western practices to bring the best of both worlds to cancer treatment. Dr. Bao completed her medical training at Johns Hopkins Medicine and joined MSKCC in 2014. Since then, she has treated hundreds of patients and helped build an integrative-medicine program that now provides services to nearly 10 percent of the institution's patients.

What is complementary and integrative medicine? How does that differ from alternative medicine?

Complementary medicine is usually nonpharmacological approaches patients use along with conventional care, such as lifestyle changes, dietary supplements, acupuncture, massage, etc. Integrative medicine refers to more evidenced-based approaches, meaning they have been shown in rigorous clinical trials to offer significant potential benefits, with low risk. As the name implies, integrative medicine (IM) is woven into and is a part of the conventional care plan.

Alternative medicine is very different because it refers to approaches patients use *instead* of conventional care, and may actually be harmful. These methods lack evidence that

continued

they work and may allow cancer to progress. Recent studies have shown that the risk of death from cancer is twice as high for patients using alternative medicine than for those receiving conventional treatment. In addition, because of the lack of evidence proving their effectiveness, these treatments usually are not covered by insurance and may be quite expensive. Often people are drawn to anecdotal incidents of people being cured from alternative treatment because they are afraid of conventional treatment. But alternative medicine does not cure cancer.

What are the main benefits of complementary/integrative care for cancer patients? How does it contribute to their well-being?

Symptom control is the main benefit. A number of complementary and integrative medicine approaches have been found to reduce the side effects of cancer and its treatment. Pain, chemotherapy-induced neuropathy, nausea and vomiting, fatigue, insomnia, joint pain from aromatase inhibitors, hot flashes, lymphedema, anxiety, and overall quality of life can all be addressed through integrative medicine. And for patients with head and neck cancers who receive chemoradiation that affects the salivary glands, IM can reduce dry mouth. These are the most common indications to use integrative medicine.

While each treatment type offers benefits against a different set of symptoms, acupuncture is among the most effective for reducing pain, hot flashes (which some breast cancer survivors experience from treatment), chemo-induced nausea, and fatigue, which is quite common among cancer survivors.

Why does acupuncture work? What is known about how it helps?

Acupuncture is a traditional Chinese medicine treatment involving the insertion of fine, single-use, sterile needles in defined acupoints. The most widely accepted theory of how it works is that neurohormonal pathways are activated by the insertion of the microthin needles. This stimulates certain nerves and sends a signal to the brain. Studies using functional MRI tests show that the central nervous system responds by releasing beta-endorphins and other neurohormones, which improve mood and decrease pain.

Acupuncture also appears to have an effect on cytokines, which are proteins released in the body to enable communication between cells, particularly in the immune system. Decreases in certain cytokines, particularly IL-6, contribute to inflammation and fatigue. Acupuncture and its corollary, acupressure, help reduce IL-6 and therefore, inflammation and fatigue.

Acupuncture is one of the most studied integrative-medicine modalities, and there is lots of evidence that it works. In addition, cancer patients are interested in using acupuncture to help alleviate pain. Among cancer survivors experiencing chronic pain, 25 percent prefer medication, 25 percent prefer acupuncture, and the rest have no preference,

continued

suggesting that acupuncture is a reasonable pain-reduction option in addition to conventional pain treatment.

Women taking aromatase inhibitors to prevent the recurrence of breast cancer have found that acupuncture reduces joint pain and stiffness. In a recent randomized controlled trial comparing acupuncture to sham acupuncture or no treatment, acupuncture significantly reduced the most-severe pain compared to sham and no acupuncture, and provided overall reduction in pain and stiffness. Acupuncture has also been shown to be as effective as the gold-standard treatment for insomnia, CBT, in cancer survivors with moderate to severe insomnia.

That said, it is not for everyone. In the clinic, about 60 to 80 percent of patients respond to treatment, not 100 percent. And it may not be appropriate for all patients. If your immune system is severely suppressed due to cancer or its treatment, the needles may pose a risk that outweighs the benefits. Additionally, some patients have needle phobia and are already being stuck so often as part of their conventional treatment that acupressure may be a better approach.

Acupressure is very similar to acupuncture, but it uses consistent pressure on specific points. An added benefit of acupressure is that once you learn it, you can do it yourself, rather than being treated by certified acupuncturists. This makes it very effective self-care. Studies have shown its effectiveness with a variety of symptoms, especially nausea and vomiting, and fatigue.

The biggest barrier to using acupuncture and acupressure is knowledge—people don't know what they are or understand how they can help. (Expense may be another barrier, as not all insurance plans cover treatment despite strong evidence demonstrating effectiveness.)

In addition to acupuncture, what are the treatment methods that you integrate into patient care to support well-being?

Diet, exercise, and mind/body approaches can benefit nearly everyone, and acupressure is helpful for many patients. In addition, I often recommend selective use of dietary supplements, expressive writing—a type of emotional detox—and massage.

What evidence do we have that these treatment modalities work?

Data on the effectiveness of a healthy **diet** is primarily from epidemiologic studies. These studies show that the Mediterranean, plant-based, and low-sugar diets can be helpful in preventing and reducing the recurrence of cancer. The evidence is moderately strong, although there have been very few controlled studies with people randomized to different diets, so it's hard to pull apart diet from other factors. That said, there is no harm attached to eating well. We have stronger evidence that low–red meat diets correlate with a lower risk for colorectal and other cancers. The more red meat one eats, the higher the incidence of colorectal cancer.

There also are so many studies about **exercise**. It wins

continued

in every aspect. It makes you feel better, decreases pain, especially aromatase-inhibitor-induced joint pain, and reduces weight, inflammation, fatigue, and overall risk of cancer and its recurrence. It also helps strengthen muscles and bones and improves body image after treatment. The evidence is pretty robust, showing minimal side effects and significant benefits.

Mind/body approaches, including meditation, yoga, and prayer, are very effective. There is strong evidence showing they reduce stress, which not only helps patients feel better but seems to reduce their risk of recurrence and helps them live longer with no side effects. Mind/body approaches are also great for reducing anxiety. Through MRI studies, we can see how meditation calms the mind and changes the pattern of brain waves. There is also a growing body of evidence that shows yoga helps with insomnia and may even help with neuropathy.

Expressive writing is another modality I recommend for most patients. [The University of Texas] MD Anderson [Cancer Center] did a large study that randomized patients with kidney cancer to either expressive writing, which meant writing their deepest thoughts and feeling about cancer, or neutral writing, and found that the group that did expressive writing felt better for longer than the narrative group. Expressive writing was shown to reduce cancer-related symptoms and improved physical functioning and possibly fatigue in patients undergoing treatment. So I recommend that my patients journal, journal, journal—try to write it all out. Think of it as an emotional detox; the way exercise is a physical detox. It helps us process our emotions and build a narrative that can help us make sense of the experience.

Patients often ask about **dietary supplements**, and overall, the evidence supporting this practice is weak. There is some evidence American ginseng can reduce fatigue, but there is also some concern about how much estrogen is in ginseng. This is particularly important for patients with hormone-sensitive cancers. In Germany, mistletoe is considered a standard of care, but not so here. There is some research to suggest it may help stimulate the immune system and reduce the side effects of chemotherapy, but the evidence is not conclusive. And what research has been done is not on oral supplements, but primarily on subcutaneous use, which has not been approved by the FDA here in the United States. Another supplement that is getting a lot of attention these days is CBD oil, and there are some data to suggest it helps with nausea, appetite, pain, and sleep, but its effectiveness is limited, and mingled with the risk of containing the psychotropic agent THC. One patient of mine reported using CBD oil to help her sleep the night before a job interview and found she just didn't feel like herself in the morning and wished she hadn't. It's not for everyone and should be used with caution.

There are also several varieties of mushrooms, including reishi mushrooms, that are taken in Asia to support long life and strength. People are now trying to extrapolate their benefit to cancer care, and while some small clinical trials suggest these traditional mushroom supplements may help increase energy and reduce fatigue, we don't know yet if they will prove useful.

continued

The most important thing with herbal supplements is that they have the potential to interfere with conventional care, so it is essential that patients check with their doctors before taking them. And if their doctors are not familiar with the potential interactions, they can always check our website or consult with us.

Most people enjoy getting a **massage**, but it actually helps with certain side effects. Not only does it help reduce stress and manage the side effects of surgery and chemotherapy, but it can help with postoperative muscle tightness, lymphedema, and chronic fatigue. There have been a number of studies done on massage, and the benefit is real, but we don't know if it sticks with you in the long-term. Without these long-term studies, most insurance companies don't cover it, so financial toxicity is a real side effect for many patients.

Which treatments can help patients address anxiety, particularly about scans and testing time?

Up to 70 percent of patients experience anxiety after a cancer diagnosis. It's hard to avoid, particularly at test time. The most-effective methods of managing anxiety in the long-term are mind/body approaches, particularly meditation, and for religious patients, prayer. I also recommend expressive writing. By keeping a journal of your cancer emotions, you can help articulate how you feel and let go of some of those emotions. And if you journal first, it makes it much easier to meditate or pray. It's also helpful to remember that there are things in life that are beyond our control—that cancer is not your fault. This is very hard for some patients.

If anxiety is particularly high, such as the night before a scan, I recommend short-term use of prescription antianxiety medication. It will help you get a better night's sleep, which makes everything better. Talk to your doctor about your anxiety and how best to manage it given your condition and treatment.

When can patients incorporate these treatments into their care?

Ideally, patients would inquire about integrative medicine when they first receive a diagnosis—there is no need to have a treatment plan in place first. Some of these things, such as diet, exercise, and meditation can even prevent cancer, so it is helpful to think about integrative medicine even before becoming a patient.

What conversations do patients need to have with their oncology care teams before initiating treatment with complementary and integrative care?

The most important thing is to let your doctors know what complementary and integrative treatments you are or want to be using. Oncologists are familiar with many of these treatments and can help you integrate them into your care, specific to your cancer and your symptoms. But if they are

continued

unfamiliar with a particular treatment or herbal supplement, they can contact an integrative medicine specialist who will help them understand if it is appropriate. Everyone can do meditation and yoga, although there may be certain poses that should be avoided because of your particular health needs. By talking to your doctor, you can determine what is right for you. Your oncologist will also know if your white blood cell count is high enough for acupuncture. Many oncologists will suggest complementary and integrative care, but if your doctor doesn't bring it up, be sure to ask.

How can patients help themselves if their hospital doesn't provide such services or they can't afford acupuncture treatment, exercise classes, or supplements?

If your oncologist okays the use of acupuncture, make sure you find a reputable provider who is familiar with acupuncture for cancer treatment. Similarly, find a yoga studio and instructor who have worked with cancer patients before. Not all yoga classes are alike, and you may want to start with gentle or restorative yoga rather than a power-flow class.

There are many meditation apps available for your phone, or you could use the resources on our website to meditate (www.mskcc.org/meditation). There is also a directory of herbs and supplements on our website and as a phone app that will tell you what is known about the effectiveness of each one. Lastly, the National Institutes of Health has a terrific site on complementary and integrative health with lots of information and resources (https://nccih.nih.gov/health).

6

HERE WE GO AGAIN: PROGRESSION AND RECURRENCE

"We must let go of the life we have planned, so as to accept the one that is waiting for us."

—*Joseph Campbell*

Unfortunately, sometimes treatment fails, and the cancer comes back. And sometimes, a second cancer emerges on the heels of—or long after—the first cancer has exacted its price. Recurrence rates vary widely, based on the type of cancer, the stage when first diagnosed, treatment, and overall patient health, from single-digit frequencies for estrogen-sensitive breast cancer treated with letrozole to a nearly universal recurrence for glioblastoma.[1] Sometimes it's the rare cancers for which there is less research and fewer treatment options that rebound, but other times, it is the common cancers—breast, prostate, colon, lung—that refuse to stay gone. Additionally, 8 to 10 percent of cancer patients develop a second cancer, or even multiple cancers, with those treated for bladder cancer and Non-Hodgkin's lymphoma, and those with certain genetic mutations, at highest risk.[2]

Regardless of the cancer or the interval between the completion of treatment and the receipt of more bad news, the blow is especially hard. The stress and anxiety that are typical with a first diagnosis are amplified as patients fear they won't ever be free of the disease. Many struggle to find hope after learning that their bodies betrayed them yet again, and feel the failure of misplaced trust in science, doctors, their faith, even themselves. Others find comfort in having had the strength to get through it once before, and rely on that strength and knowledge to tackle a return engagement. But it is a difficult time for all, evoking a complex range of emotions.

From Disappointment to Devastation

Michael was disillusioned when his colorectal cancer recurred ten years after it was first treated. Not only was the cancer in a more challenging location, necessitating aggressive surgery that included the removal of two-thirds of his stomach, but the physical challenges were compounded by the emotional ones.

> It was a huge emotional blow. I felt disappointment and was so fearful. I had learned from my first experience with cancer that I could survive, and this time I had my girlfriend at my side saying, "We will deal with it," so I didn't feel alone. But it was still so

hard. I had to learn to study my options, accept the doctor's advice, and trust spiritually that I was being cared for.

Now I'm more appreciative of every single day. I know cancer can come back at any time, but I'm going to live fully. Some things I can't control, but I can control how I feel about them. I suspect that cancer will come back in some form again, but I try not to obsess about it.

Recurrence is a common theme for women with ovarian cancer. While many women are cured after their initial treatment, as many as 85 percent have a second or third recurrence,[3] despite having a full remission after their first diagnosis and treatment. (Note: these data relate to historic rates as of 2019 and do not reflect current treatment protocols since the addition of immunotherapy, poly ADP ribose polymerase [PARP] inhibitors, PD-1 inhibitors, and other new therapies. Your prognosis may be different.) The cancer remains dormant for months or even years at a time, reemerging to bring physical and emotional turmoil yet again. Anger often accompanies the fear, particularly after a difficult return to health the first time. As Anne said after her first recurrence, "I don't think I have ever been so angry." But she was also disappointed in herself and in her medical team.

I felt like a complete failure and felt that everyone was so tired of me and my cancer. What was all that heroism the first time even for? I really dislike the "win the battle" language, but it's hard not to feel as though you are a loser when it comes back.

The third recurrence came right on the heels of the second, and I thought I was going to die. I was terrified, really scared, but I also began to think that this was really just a part of my life now, and that I needed to accept it.

Evolving from thinking of cancer as an acute disease to seeing it as one that is chronic and needs to be managed also helps patients deal with the disappointment and anger. As Sue M., a psychologist and mother of three who received her first diagnosis of ovarian cancer at age fifty, explained after her third recurrence, "We all wish to have some control over the circumstances of our lives, but of course we cannot."

I was completely devastated all over again when it came back a third time. How could this be happening again? And why? I was ready to spin out of control, but then my doctor helped me change my mindset. He emphasized that we really need to think of it as a chronic condition. So I am recalibrating.

I have moments of calm, but the cancer is always with me. I worry about it all the time. I'm trying hard to keep a clear mind about it and to engage with life, but it's challenging. With every random symptom, I have to ask myself, "Is it a torn ligament or is it coming back?" I don't take the future for granted. But I'm sitting here with a full head of hair and the assurance that everything is going to be okay because they caught it early.

When it came back the first time, I didn't tell anyone. I didn't want people to think of me as a cancer patient. Now I recognize that I am a cancer patient, but in a different category. I kind of want people to catch up with the idea of chronic cancer. I am a cancer patient, and I am always somewhat vulnerable.

Some people find that the news of recurrence loses its sting over time. As with controlled-exposure therapy for phobias and PTSD, each recurrence and recovery helps them build confidence that the next hurdle can also be overcome, and so a new diagnosis loses some of its emotional power. As Deborah made clear after her fifth recurrence of ovarian cancer and eighty-eight chemo infusions over fifteen years, "It's just gotten so old, to the point where I feel like, 'Oh, ho hum, it is what it is.'

> Now, at seventy-eight, something is going to take me pretty soon; it might as well be cancer. But I am more worried about being killed in the car getting to the hospital for appointments! At the time of my first recurrence, my doctor said, "You will never be completely free of cancer, so we will treat it like a chronic disease. It will flare up, we will treat it, it will go away, and if it comes back, we will do it again." That was very reassuring, so I didn't freak out when it came back again and again.

Against the Odds

Sometimes one cancer diagnosis leads to another, different cancer as a result of a genetic predisposition, prior treatment, or just plain bad luck. And when that second cancer can't be easily tamed, a return engagement brings anger, frustration, even rage, as Jim experienced after his second diagnosis with thyroid cancer.

> At first I thought, "We beat this once, we will beat it again; what's the big deal?" But I later learned it wasn't that my cancer had come back. Instead, it was a second type of rare cancer that probably grew alongside the first and remained hidden because it doesn't respond to the usual treatment. And since there was no thyroid left, it migrated to my lungs.
>
> Once I understood that and was told to put my affairs in order, I was angry. I ranted for the whole drive home. "Why me? How can they be so sure? What's going to happen to my kids? I won't get to see my grandkids." All those thoughts and emotions ran through me. And I am still angry. It's an ongoing issue.
>
> At four years in, I am one of the longest-surviving patients with this type of cancer, but we have shot two of the three magic bullets against this rare disease, and the tumors in my lungs are still growing. So my anger continues. It seems anger is my normal response to getting disappointed. So I am seeking to replace that disappointment with the hope and peace that comes from knowing Jesus.

Having people who depend on you can heighten the sense of urgency with a second diagnosis. Christina, a yoga instructor who owned her own studio until she had breast cancer at age forty-eight, discovered this the hard way when she was diagnosed with esophageal cancer just as she was finishing treatment for her first cancer.

> When I heard my oncologist say, "I cured you of breast cancer, but this is different; put your affairs in order," it was really intense. It's terrifying facing your mortality when you have two young kids at home. I have to be there for my kids, have to see them through high school and college.
>
> When I wake up in the morning, before my feet touch the floor, I remember, "Oh yes, I am still dealing with cancer, and might be dealing with it for the rest of my life—it might be a very long life, but I don't know." I get really sad. It's exhausting, but I need to honor the feelings of sadness and fear and deal with the unknown. And I need to get well so I can take care of my kids.

The long-term ramifications of multiple cancers can be complex, as Angela learned. She had cervical cancer at age twenty-five and discovered after her third cancer at age forty-one that she had a mutation of a gene that helps control tumor growth, making her susceptible to a variety of cancers.

> Going through cancer so many times is bad enough, but the fallout from cancer and treatment is even worse. I don't have active disease right now, but I haven't found a way to feel close to where I was before, physically or emotionally. I've got neuropathy from the chemo and nerve damage from the

surgeries. I'm in constant pain, and on pain medication that has affected my independence. I had to stop driving, I'm sleepy, forgetful, and just not able to function at the same capacity as before. I couldn't go back to a job that demands political sensitivity, swiftness, and full mental focus.

The physical changes lead right into emotional ones. When I stopped working and officially left my job, my identity in the family as the problem solver and breadwinner stopped. I loved being that person and feel as if my family doesn't look at me the same way anymore. They don't come to me for advice and input, even on things that affect me, which is so disrespectful and condescending.

On top of all that, the radiation for my cervical cancer caused colon issues, so I have a colostomy. It's a visual, daily reminder of how cancer has never really left me. It's hard to manage the self-identity issues that creates. Just try to feel sexy with a bag of poop hanging off you!

SCIENCE SIDEBAR: DEALING WITH CANCER PAIN

Pain is a common experience in cancer. As many as 50 percent of patients undergoing treatment experience some type of pain, increasing to 70 to 90 percent of those with advanced disease.[4] The pain may be caused by the cancer itself or be a side effect of treatment, and often doesn't resolve even after treatment has ended.

The type and severity of pain vary significantly by cancer location and stage, as well as by treatment, but can include pain from tumors pressing on organs, tissue, and bone; from tumor invasion of bone or organs increasing pressure from within; from nerve damage caused by tumors themselves; or as a direct result of surgery, neurotoxic chemotherapy, or radiation. Surgery can be a direct cause of pain, both at the incision site and due to nerve injury. And surgical complications, such as infection or the development of thick scar tissue, can also contribute to discomfort, as can the swelling and lymphedema that sometimes result from surgery.

Radiation can cause swelling, tenderness, and skin burns, all of which hurt, and chemo and immunotherapy can cause a variety of ailments, including damage to mucus membranes (typically experienced as mouth sores), gastrointestinal distress, general muscle and bone achiness, and headache. And let's not forget the frequent needle sticks and injections and even lumbar punctures for monitoring the disease and administering treatment. When all goes well, they last but a moment, but it's not unusual, particularly after repeated

continued

treatments, for the care team to struggle to find a vein or to place a venous catheter, resulting in chemo drugs leaking into sensitive tissue.

Many patients experience multiple types of pain in one or more locations. For instance, a tumor on an ovary may put pressure on the spine and be felt as a dull backache, while one pressing on the intestine may cause severe stomach cramps. At the same time, the chemo cocktail used to treat ovarian (and many other types of) cancer may induce peripheral neuropathy, which is experienced as a numbness and tingling or even burning pain in the hands and feet.

In addition to the physical sensations caused by the presence of a tumor, its growth can change the chemical balance in tissue surrounding the tumor, increasing the release of histamines, cytokines, prostaglandins, and other mediators of pain.[5] This turns up the body's sensitivity to the physical presence of the tumor, and increases pain. It also contributes to fatigue, another multiplier of pain.[6]

Dealing with this pain becomes part of the cancer ordeal, heightening the anxiety about treatment and adding to the trauma of the experience. With each recurrence or new diagnosis, patients anticipate the recurrence of pain, initiating a stress reaction that further heightens their sensitivity to pain. This pain and the anxiety it causes have a significant impact on patients, compromising their quality of life while they are undergoing treatment and thereafter, and unfortunately, can interfere with the completion of treatment. Women stop taking their aromatase inhibitors due to bone pain, despite recommendations to continue for five or even ten years.

Patients discontinue immunotherapy regimens when their mouth sores interfere with their ability to eat.

In most cases, patients can achieve substantial relief from pain if they voice their concerns. Doses can be adjusted, pain medication and complementary therapies can be added to the regimen, and treatment plans can be changed. But not all doctors seem receptive to hearing about pain, and patients often feel that they should just "suck it up" and suffer through it. Forty percent of patients being treated in community-based hospitals don't feel they receive the desired advice and help for their pain.[7] While many large hospitals and cancer centers have supportive-care practices that include pain management, particularly for inpatient care, outpatient supportive care is less common, and smaller hospitals may not provide this service at all.

Reducing your physical pain can improve your quality of life and help you cope with your disease and treatment. Talk to your doctor about your pain and other symptoms. Your oncologist may be able to address your needs directly or refer you to supportive-care colleagues on her team. If not, patients in most communities can access pain-management and supportive-care services through external providers. (The Center to Advance Palliative Care— getpalliativecare.org—has a provider directory organized by zip code. Note: palliative care does not mean hospice care. It means making it better. To palliate is to alleviate or ease, and does not mean giving up on treatment, a common misperception.) And check with your insurance plan regarding coverage. Most insurance plans, including Medicare and

continued

Medicaid, will pay for management of pain and other symptoms, although Medicaid varies by state. Your hospital social worker or financial counselor may also be able to help you access symptom-management care if funding is an issue.

Diagnosis Foretold

Perhaps the most disheartening news for a person with a history of cancer is that treatment received in the course of recovering from an earlier diagnosis has led to a second cancer. This was certainly the case for Steve, who was diagnosed with testicular cancer at age thirty. At the time, he was warned that radiation therapy might lead to a second cancer. But a diagnosis of stage 4 colon cancer at fifty-five was not what he anticipated.

> I always knew I would get cancer again, and have been watching and keeping an eye on the clock. But I assumed it would be much later. I knew nothing about colon cancer and had an immediate fear of my mortality. When I heard the news, I didn't think "Okay, no problem, let's just fight it." No, it was more like, "Oh crap, this is the beginning of the end." I started thinking about everything I needed to do to wrap things up. And my first thought was who was going to take care of my dogs? I have six dogs. No one can step in and take care of six dogs.
>
> My doctor hasn't offered any numbers on my likely survival, but he thinks I am responding well to treatment, and the most recent scan was good.

I don't know what the endgame is going to be. I'm just taking it one day at a time.

Fran, who is on her third cancer, is also focused on getting back to normal, whatever that might be. Diagnosed with chronic myelogenous leukemia at age forty-nine, Fran had chemotherapy and full-body radiation in preparation for a bone-marrow transplant in 1995. Her healthy "new normal" lasted until 2003 when she relapsed. Fortunately, by then a new drug was available that put her in remission, and she remained healthy for the next thirteen years. But the radiation she had in preparation for the transplant is a known risk for subsequent cancers and in 2016 she was diagnosed with breast cancer that required a mastectomy, followed six months later with a diagnosis of urothelial cancer, making "normal" even harder to attain.

I was so shocked and angry that the bone-marrow transplant had failed after eight years. It had taken so much out of me and put me at increased risk for future problems. At the time, I had thought maybe skin cancer or cataracts, both of which I subsequently had, but not urothelial cancer. I was lucky and not so worried about the breast cancer— it was my quality of life that was compromised, not a death sentence. But this latest diagnosis feels especially ominous. It's a cancer that could kill me.

At seventy-five, my body is less resilient. The cancer has persisted despite removal of a kidney and a year of standard and experimental treatments. Now I'm on a relatively new drug for metastatic cancer. Managing the side effects is the biggest challenge.

The drug will not cure me, but is extending my life. For that I am grateful, as well as for the love and support of my amazing husband.

It doesn't help to be depressed and hopeless, although I can't always avoid it. I'm trying not to think about death and to enjoy life as much as I can, including playing tennis when I have the energy! It's not easy. However, when I do think and talk about death, I find it comforting."

Many patients with secondary or recurrent cancers recover again and go on to live long and healthy lives. The mechanisms that allowed for the return engagement may not be any more threatening than the initial cancer, even if it feels otherwise. Anne has been free of ovarian cancer for twelve years and believes she is done. Jennifer's third cancer was dispatched with barely a wrinkle in her daily life, and Deborah's usually able to forget she is a cancer patient, despite having been one for twenty-two years.

But others are not so fortunate, and the recurrence actually represents a progression, a sign of the body's inability to clear an ever more wily and invasive disease. Cancer that has metastasized to the lungs, bone, or brain will be much harder to eliminate, and many of these patients will never fully recover, despite some living longer than anticipated. As Eileen, who had recurrent breast cancer before being diagnosed with metastatic mesothelioma, said, "No one expected me to still be around so long after this diagnosis. I know one woman who lived fourteen years with the disease. I don't think I will last that long, but I figure I've got another year or two. So I just keep getting on with life."

ADVICE FROM THOSE WHO
LEARNED IT THE HARD WAY

While dealing with recurrence or disease progression is never easy, a few themes emerge from those who have been there. They focus on how you think about your own situation and how you guide others to think about and communicate with you.

As Fran said, it helps to be in the moment. "Try not to think about the 'what if's. Don't deny reality, but don't focus on it either. Instead, try to get out and be with friends." Michael agreed. "Just take one day at a time. Focus on happiness and stay positive."

Sue M. echoed that idea. "Try to do things to help stay calm—meditate, walk the dog, go for a run. Having a meditation practice really helps. I've come to understand the crucial importance of mindset, mindfulness, and gratitude as coping skills for all realms of life. I am increasingly convinced that how we perceive our reality is how we live our reality."

Recognizing that some things are out of your hands also helps. Jim said, "There is no such thing as control, so try to live on what you know, not what you don't know. As devastating as this diagnosis has been, the first place I go emotionally is to my relationship with God." Eileen also advised faith. "Facing mortality will frighten us all. You need something to help you transcend it. Religion or faith in something that goes beyond the material can help you find the strength to get through it. There are spiritual resources out there to help."

Angela also found that having faith can be a source of strength. "I have faith in God, and lately have started believing in myself again too. What really got me through this is remembering that I am smart and brave, and knowing that while God is going to be there for me, I can figure things out and do the best I can for myself. Of course, it also helps to have a good friend I can talk to and cry with."

Deborah agreed. "Depend on the people around you. Don't be afraid to share it. So many people don't want to talk about it, but I think it is important that you allow people in. It makes it a lot less scary. You don't have to feel that people are intruding, but don't try to do it all yourself. There are so many people who care." Nancy I. said, "I found an online support group for my specific cancer and it has helped in lots of ways. There is so much information and support there. I even learn things my doctor doesn't know."

Christina also recommended seeking support. "Find your support system, whatever it may be, and use it. People want to connect to what is real at the end of the day. They may want reassurance from you that you are going to be fine, but they also want to help. It gives them a sense of purpose. Give those who love you and care about you a chance to help. It creates a virtuous circle that is bound to help you feel loved at a difficult time."

But Anne warned, "It's so important to educate people not to toss off scary predictions about your future. I would love to see caregivers and friends develop an awareness that the patient isn't telling you everything. They are probably way more scared than they want to put on you, so don't make it worse."

END OF LIFE: DENIAL, ANGER, AND FACING THE INEVITABLE

"Every man must do two things alone; he must do his own believing and his own dying."

—*Martin Luther*

While mortality rates continue to decline, thanks to a decrease in smoking, earlier detection of several malignancies, and some improvement in treatments, cancer still claims the lives of more than 600,000 people each year in the United States alone.[1] One-third of those receiving a cancer diagnosis will succumb to the disease within five years. But within that number, there is huge variation, based on type of disease, patient health at the time of diagnosis, how advanced the cancer is when discovered, and the quality and timing of treatment.[2]

For those unlucky enough to be on the wrong end of the statistical distribution, the inevitability of dying from cancer can be challenging to accept. Most cancer deaths are not sudden, giving patients and their loved ones a chance to get adjusted to the idea. But often, patients feel relatively healthy and independent until a precipitous decline in the final three to four months of life.[3] This apparent healthiness can make it easy for patients and their loved ones to deny destiny. Acceptance becomes a slow process, a gradual shifting in expectations and assumptions, or even an iterative bargain.

Sometimes, patients with a new diagnosis will maintain hopefulness in spite of a grim prognosis. David, a retired writer and editor who was diagnosed with acute myeloid leukemia (AML) just weeks after moving across the country to be with "the love of his life," knew early on that the diagnosis was devastating. He was in and out of the hospital multiple times over the course of a few months, even marrying his love while there for one extended stay, but remained optimistic that he would make a full recovery despite the odds.

It's hard to look death in the eye. It's scary and sad. I feel that if I die in the near future, I'm going to miss out on a lot of things that would be pleasurable if I am around to do them. I feel even sadder for the people I'm leaving. A few will be devastated.

But it is what it is. There is nothing to be done about it—it's a fact that I have AML. I don't see the point of not dealing with it. You could say I'm just whistling past the graveyard here and acting as if everything is good. I know what diagnosis I've got, and that the prognosis is not great. Still, I'm healthy and fit, and if anyone is going to be equipped to beat a disease like this, it's me.

But often, time provides the opportunity to begin a process of acceptance. Paul lived for ten years with a neuroendocrine cancer that gradually took over his life. A former pharmacist with a black belt in judo, he went, as his disease progressed, from total disbelief to recognition that his days were numbered.

> I thought I had appendicitis or something. I couldn't believe when they said it was cancer. My wife said I was stuttering when they told me the news. I have had enough relatives die of cancer to know what that means. Intellectually, I know that cancer doesn't have to be a death sentence, but emotionally....
>
> The gradual loss of independence, of being able to do things for myself, has really been hard. I gave up driving ten years ago, stopped working three years ago. I have near-constant abdominal pain, diarrhea, and bone thinning, which has taken judo away from me altogether—I can't take a fall. And there is tremendous depression that goes along with this, in part from the alternated lifestyle, but mainly from the chemical imbalance caused by the disease.
>
> The depression has really affected me. I know that at some point, this disease does so much damage that you die. There are days when I get into my chair in the den and don't move other than to run to the bathroom. It's put a strain on my relationship. Libby said this changes nothing between us, but I'm

a tremendous burden on her. Even as recently as two years ago, I did most of the cooking, but now, eating isn't something I like.

It's surprising how quickly things are changing now. Every day is so unpredictable. It's unsettling because I feel as though there is nothing I can do. It's not like prepping for a competition or even rehabbing a knee, both of which I have done plenty of times. You can't prep for a cancer death; there are no muscles you can train. You can't overcome it by pushing your body to the limit. I am beyond the limit already.

Changing expectations and increasing understanding of the reality of her situation is part of Carol's experience too. Diagnosed with stage 4 uterine cancer, she has undergone surgery, radiation, and chemotherapy to control the cancer, with limited success.

I guess I sort of assumed that things were going to be okay. But at one point, my doctor said he didn't want to see me for three months. I asked if that meant that I was in remission and he said, "What part of stage 4 cancer don't you understand?" I haven't asked many questions after that. His comment just stuck a knife in it. Now I go from one scan to the next. If I get a clean scan, I take on the next project. That's the way I've been living my life for the last three years. I hope I get a few more because I still have a lot of things to do in order to get things ready for when I'm gone.

For many patients coming to terms with impending death, preparing for their own absence is part of the process. Taking care of loved ones, cleaning up messes, setting the record straight—it's not unusual for patients to use the time to ensure that they don't leave behind any unfinished business.

Jeremy had officially retired from the military shortly before his cancer was discovered. Because the symptoms were nonspecific, and the cancer (pseudomyxoma peritonei) was so rare, it had already progressed to stage 4 before he was diagnosed and treated. He had massive surgery and aggressive chemo to clear the disease. Then, eight months later, the real bad news came.

> My cancer was back. When I heard that, all I could think of was this was some sort of BS. "What do you mean, it's back?" I was supposed to have eleven years still [to reach the average life expectancy after diagnosis], and now those eleven years were looking pretty good. All the data show that when it comes back right away, 80 to 90 percent of patients are dead within five years. So now I know I am going to die, and not when I'm eighty. I'm just trying to figure out how to get to fifty. I want to see my kids through college, but I don't want to die then either, because I don't want my wife to be alone.
>
> I saw a psychiatrist right after the recurrence. I cried for forty-five minutes in his office about all the crap that isn't fair. My life isn't over but the reality of being told nothing is going to stop my cancer messes with my head.
>
> I have learned that I don't have to beat cancer, I just have to get through it. I just have to deal with

it one day at a time. I don't dwell on death, but I do think about it every day, sometimes multiple times a day. I'm in no hurry to die, but I don't want to feel bad either. I want my old self back, but that's just not going to happen.

There are times I think I would rather just die than go through another day of this crap, but I want to make sure my sons understand certain things I won't be around to explain to them later. And I want to make sure my wife and kids will be cared for when I'm gone. So I keep pushing.

Unfortunately, intellectually understanding your path doesn't make it any easier to find emotional acceptance. Robert, a seventy-four-year-old former economist and passionate artist who had been battling pancreatic cancer for two years, began receiving hospice care at home. He knew his time was near. "What mostly affected me was not the strong desire that overwhelmed me to get in the studio and paint again, but the realization that that may never happen. I remained detached from all this and accepted it," he said. But wrapping up a busy life is a messy process.

I have been going through a cleansing phase, throwing out all kinds of old papers and things from my office. Yesterday I deleted almost two thousand emails. I recycled maps of trails I took in the northwest and Canada when I was in my twenties. I know I will not do those hikes again.

In my quest to clear my desk, I came across an article on death and dying I had torn out a year or so back. It wrote of the failure of the body as the end of life approaches. There were three charts. One showed a steady decline, getting a little weaker each day until the end; another showed a more stable life and then a more abrupt decline; and the third showed a decline in fits and starts, alternating between stability and decline. But none of the charts showed any improvement at any time, just a change in the decline rate.

I am starting to take this all in. My condition will only get worse; it is just a question of the path down. Of course, it is difficult to accept, and one can hope that this time may be different, but the better approach is acceptance, which is hard for me as well as for my wife, family, and friends.

Parallel Processing

While patients are processing their own losses, dealing with pain and coming to terms with an impending death, their loving caretakers may be struggling to accommodate to the new reality as well. Sometimes patients get there first; other times it's the family. Sometimes the patient wants to be in control; other times the patient wants the family to take over, or the family wants to keep reality from the patient as long as possible. And the situation for loving caregivers is made all the more complicated by the realities of being left behind emotionally, physically, and financially.

For Ann R., the biggest challenge was the feeling of helplessness as she watched her husband of more than fifty years, a doctor and athlete who had maintained a smoking habit for decades despite knowing every reason he shouldn't, succumb to lung cancer.

I wanted to go along with how he was feeling, which was that he would be treated and be okay, but as soon as you hear the word "cancer," your heart is in your throat—or really, in your feet. He never commented on his fate, but I was beside myself all the time.

I gave up everything that I usually did so I could take care of him. I drove him to see oncologists, neurologists, to do blood typing. I sat in hospitals and doctors' offices every single day for hours. And as he deteriorated, I pushed his wheelchair. I didn't complain. It's just what you do.

But it was hard to watch him losing weight and being so tired, losing his balance, no longer able to do his activities. Seeing the deterioration of someone you love is painful. When Bob had asked the oncologist how many years he would have and the doctor had said, "Maybe five," that got to us right away. But who knew that it wouldn't be five and that there wouldn't even be a few good years?

Because your focus is always on the patient, you don't have a chance to replenish yourself. I didn't do what I would usually do, but rather we would sit and read together, watch sports together, cook dinner, have people over to the house. And when people came over, I could leave because I knew someone was there. It allowed me to take a back seat in his care for brief times. Otherwise, I was afraid to leave the house. What if he fell or needed something and couldn't get it?

Even though I was doing all that I could for him, I felt so helpless watching his progression. It was very frustrating. There were times I felt upset about why this was happening to us, what life had given us to deal with. And once he was in the hospital, I found coming home by myself so dispiriting. I didn't want to eat, didn't want to do anything. I realized that he wasn't going to recover, that he wasn't going to get out of the hospital. But I couldn't show my grief—I had to be strong for him and the kids.

Taking responsibility for the patient and others at the expense of self is often the norm for caregivers, as Audrey learned. After having a series of seizures, her husband, Matthew, ended up in the hospital shortly after his fifty-ninth birthday. She arranged to transport him from London, where they had been living for more than a decade, to the United States for treatment for the seizures, but it was a total shock to learn that the cause of the seizures was glioblastoma. "That was just not on my radar," she said, "and when they told me that, I nearly passed out." It was also the start of a life-changing journey.

I made the determination not to tell Matthew right away. He was heavily sedated, and we took time to ease into it. While he slept, I went to work figuring out how to beat it, talking to doctors at Duke, Columbia, Mass General. The research was hard to read. No one survives.

My husband was a brilliant man, but he didn't want to hear any of it. He handed the whole thing over to me, the researching and the conversations with doctors and the responsibility. While he slept, I'd research. I became an expert in the disease, knew everything about clinical trials, drugs, etc. He had fears about what the diagnosis meant, but suppressed them. We never discussed death. He couldn't do it, which made it all the more difficult for me. I didn't sleep, couldn't let my guard down in front of him, never had any time off.

There were times when I would go to the psychologist's office and just collapse. Or when he was in the hospital, or having a seizure. It was just horrible, a real hellhole. But I never lost it in front of him. I had enough self-awareness to know that I needed to take breaks, and sometimes I would just take the dog for a walk to escape. But I had stopped life to take care of him and didn't have time to build a new one.

I felt like a refugee. We had arrived in New York with two suitcases and a dog, but it was clear we were never going back to our old lives. Once he had the glioblastoma diagnosis, we were told we were lucky if he had seven months. I was coming to terms with a lot of changes all at the same time.

While Matthew did his best to ignore the realities of his condition, burdening his wife with the decision-making, Harvey, dealing with progressive multiple myeloma, tried to maintain as much independence and control as possible, despite having a capable doctor as a wife. "He was extremely protective of me," Maria said, although she accompanied him to all his appointments.

> In the first meeting with the oncologist, the doctor told Harvey he would keep him alive until something else kills him. That was the best thing, psychologically, that anyone could have said to him.
>
> And it turned out to be right—he died of complications of the chemo. But just hearing those words helped him. He was reassured by those words and never doubted and worried.
>
> I knew that he knew he was going to die. For years we were talking about cleaning out old papers, and then, in November, he took it upon himself to do all that stuff. I think he knew he was going to die, but he didn't want to discuss it. He just did the papers. His cancer developed very slowly, so ultimately, it was not a shock.
>
> I think his whole approach to life was based on his parents' experiences as Holocaust survivors. Whatever he had to endure was nothing compared to what his parents went through, so Harvey just went with the flow. It is what it is; no use to worry ahead of time.
>
> As a spouse, [I found that] the hardest thing was the helplessness. I had the sense that there was no way to make it any better. And Harvey resented that I had to do more stuff for him. He was resigned to his illness, even though he was used to controlling everything else.

Sometimes, the more you know, the harder it is. That was certainly the case for Kevin when his wife, Donna, was diagnosed with stage 3 lung cancer. "When we got the news, I sobbed uncontrollably the whole way home," he said. "She didn't shed a single tear—assured me that it was going to be okay—but I knew it wasn't going to be." A doctor himself, he knew enough about cancer to know the prognosis wasn't good.

It was a constant struggle between hope and fear. The plans kept changing as her condition progressed more rapidly and with more complications than anyone expected. It was an iterative process of bargaining, where what you hope for changes and changes and changes again in an ongoing process of renegotiating with the possible.

At one point, about a year into the diagnosis, she was pretty sick and I didn't think she was going to live to leave the hospital. I had spent six or seven consecutive nights in the hospital and was getting loopy from lack of sleep and fear and grief. I remember saying to her sister, "I don't even know what to pray for anymore." And she wisely replied, "As many good days as possible." That was what we had come to.

In the last few weeks, she had metastases in many bones and was in a lot of pain. By then, anything that could possibly be considered a good day had disappeared. All you hope for is an easy passing. Then she was gone, leaving a void in the world for so many of us.

I had eighteen months of knowing Donna had a terminal illness before she died. You try to prepare, and you try not to prepare. Preparing is giving up; not preparing leaves you in intolerable vulnerability. Still, the hardest part was the sequential giving up of various hopes—that it's not cancer, that surgery and long-term remission are possible, that she will have a lot of good days, that she won't suffer too much—that war of sequential compromise, bargains made, lost, remade, and ultimately the recognition that reprieve is impossible. There would be no reprieve. She greatly outlived her prognosis, but I knew her illness was a death sentence and the inevitable is coming, came, has passed.

Randi had a similar sense of having tried repeatedly to outsmart her husband's cancer. A nurse by training, she knew from the beginning that a diagnosis of glioblastoma would not end well. "In the end, his body foiled my great attempt to save him. It was so hard coming to terms with what's possible versus not possible, not in my control. That the disease is more powerful than the most powerful love between two people. But the adjustment to reality takes time."

You don't stop breathing when something like that happens. You are still there, and you have to do what you have to do. I had to be there for the kids. If not, I think it would have been hard to get out of bed. Even the older two in college, they still needed me. I told them we were all going on with our lives, as Daddy would have wanted. Another dear friend gave them their marching orders in his powerful eulogy. I wanted them in therapy and back in school so that they could get on with their lives. For close to a year, I would cry every night. And when I had finally fallen asleep, I would wake up crying the next morning.

I went to the therapist fourteen days after he died, I cried and cried. After two hours he asked, "Are you wearing underwear?" I couldn't imagine why that was relevant, but when I said yes, he said, "Then you are doing very well." I laugh now, but when I look back, I realize that I had more strength than I ever imagined. I would have thought I couldn't handle it or manage anything afterward, but I did. There were always two voices in my head—"I can't do this" and "I have to do this." I would get up in the morning and make the bed right away, just to show myself that I was functioning.

SCIENCE SIDEBAR: HOW WE DIE FROM CANCER

The majority of patients who die from end-stage cancer experience progressive fatigue, shortness of breath, drowsiness, feeling unwell, and lack of appetite in the final weeks of life,[4] and many slip into a coma before actually dying of multiorgan failure. Typically, the disease starts the process by causing some local organ damage, which affects homeostasis—the body's natural balancing act—and precipitates a general decline. The location of the primary cancer usually drives the particular organ first involved. For instance, colon and other cancers in the abdomen may damage the liver, which will cause the liver to stop clearing toxins from the body, inducing liver coma. And when the digestive tract is invaded, the reduced capacity for normal intake of nourishment leads to kidney failure, which typically progresses to brain failure due to the accumulation of toxins in the brain.[5] Or if the lungs are involved, there may not be enough oxygen circulating, which leads to an accumulation of carbon dioxide and also progresses to brain failure.

Most people enter into a drowsy state a few days before dying and many lose conscious awareness of their physical suffering.[6] Breathing becomes more irregular—for some, more rapid and superficial, while others take deep, intermittent breaths—as progressive damage in the brain interferes with normal breathing reflexes. Although many patients experience pain in the final months of their disease, those receiving palliative support generally have their pain and nausea well-managed in the final days preceding a coma and death.[7]

continued

Of course, there are exceptions. Some patients may have blood clots that can lead to circulatory arrest. Or their hearts may fail. Still others may develop severe infections due to suppressed immune function as a result of the disease or treatment.[8] But even these unanticipated, sudden deaths are generally experienced as comas—just sooner than anyone would have anticipated.

Some cancers have the ability to interfere more directly with the flow of oxygen, through metastases or primary cancer growth in the lungs, throat, or carotid arteries, or with the function of the brain. Typically, doctors closely monitor the progression of these cancers in order to anticipate suffering and provide palliative care in advance of discomfort. Management of anxiety, shortness of breath, and other symptoms in addition to pain is part of the supportive-care process as a patient nears the end of life.

NEARING THE END

Doctors look at a variety of factors in assessing how soon a patient may die from cancer, starting with how well a patient is functioning and what if any symptoms the patient is experiencing. There are clinical events that can indicate progression, such as acute deep-vein thrombosis, hypercalcemia, or spinal cord compression, all signs that the patient's life is wrapping up in the next couple of weeks to months. There are also serum markers of death from cancer—increased white blood cell count, decreased lymphocyte counts, increased calcium in the blood, and decreased sodium in the blood—as well as changes in key vital signs such as increased heart rate, decreased blood pressure, and lower oxygen saturation rates.[9]

But overall, the strongest predictor of death will be the functional status of the patients—if they are still dressing themselves and getting to the doctor, then they're okay. The more dependent a patient becomes on others for activities of daily living, the higher the likelihood of dying soon. A patient with stage 4 cancer who has become bedbound and dependent on others for bathroom functions, eating, dressing, and other activities of daily living rarely lives beyond six weeks.[10] That is the point at which most doctors encourage home care or hospice care. But it can be hard for a doctor to guide patients toward death when she has been fighting alongside them for so long.

And once a patient is bedbound and close to death, there are additional stages that clarify for doctors that it may be only days until the patient starts to exhibit brain failure. Typically, patients will begin to invert their sleep-wake cycles, becoming agitated at night and sleeping most of the day. In the beginning of this terminal downward slope, they may have hallucinations, be disoriented, and not recognize family members. They may not experience thirst, not urinate, and exhibit other signs of organ failure. That's when doctors can say with confidence that death is going to be in the next couple of days or couple of weeks.[11]

THE EMOTIONAL EXPERIENCE OF DEATH

While popular media sometimes refer to Elisabeth Kübler-Ross's "five stages of grief"—in which people are said to

continued

pass through emotions such as denial, anger, bargaining, depression, and finally acceptance—in reality, the emotional experience of death is neither linear nor consistent. How we respond to imminent death is influenced by our prior psychological experiences, personalities, and underlying resiliency. For many patients dying of cancer, the physical reality of remaining relatively independent for months or years in the face of a terminal diagnosis provides an opportunity either to remain in denial or to slowly prepare. And a subsequent increase in pain and decline in function in the final months often bring a desire for relief and release. As a patient's world becomes smaller, it gets harder to deny that death is imminent, and easier to accept and be grateful for it.

Unfortunately, the helplessness of loved ones often confounds that experience. Sitting on the sidelines, they see a patient go from vibrant to weak, from optimistic to accepting, and are unable to provide more than loving support while often remaining unaware of the subtle physical changes that drive this evolution.

Most people are resilient,[12] and they reach acceptance of death, either for themselves or their loved ones. But patients with higher levels of anxiety about death and its impact on others often also suffer greater feelings of demoralization, including a sense of helplessness or failure to meet their own or others' expectations. And, feeling demoralized is often associated with experiencing a greater burden of symptoms, including pain.[13] No one wants to be dependent on others, suffer, or die without dignity, and yet these concerns are often the drivers of the greatest distress when coming to terms with a cancer death.[14]

Some patients also suffer spiritual distress in their final months, unsure that they have lived up to the expectations of their faith and will find the promised peace, while others rely on their faith to help them deal with their physical and existential distress.

While there is no one-size-fits-all process for coping with the distress of terminal cancer and impending death, many hospitals and cancer centers offer supportive-care services, also called palliative care, that can help address the physical and emotional concerns of patients and loving caregivers. Everything from pain medication, massage, and complementary therapies to individual, family, and group counseling is generally available, along with experts who can lead a conversation about how the patient would like to die. Most hospitals have relationships with hospice facilities and can make arrangements for hospice at home or for hospital stays, each with the assurance of relief from pain, providing patients and their families with options for how the final days will be lived.

SIDEBAR: Q AND A ON CARING FOR PATIENTS AT THE END OF THEIR LIVES

Palliative-care doctors improve the quality of life for patients and their families by offering supportive care throughout the course of cancer to reduce pain, manage symptoms, and provide relief from the stress of living with a serious illness. But when a patient's disease no longer responds to treatment, palliative-care doctors play a specific role in helping patients make the switch from prolonging life to curtailing suffering. **Dr. Cristian Zanartu, attending physician, internist, and palliative-medicine specialist at Montefiore Medical Center** in the Bronx, New York, treats hundreds of patients a month with advanced cancer and helps prepare them for the physical and emotional issues that arise at the end of life.

When do you initiate conversations with patients about end-of-life care?

Usually, I try to start a dialogue whenever a patient is up against a big challenge, and there are two types of challenges. The first is when patients have cancers that we know are not going to go well, when the numbers are stacked against them. This is very tricky because even if the patients currently look amazing, we know this is going to change, so we want to help them think about the "what-if"s. The second type of challenge comes when a patient's disease progresses even after multiple courses of treatment. These patients, the unlucky ones who didn't respond or [couldn't] sustain a response, are likely to face the same challenge and we want them to be ready for it.

Treatment is evolving at a rapid pace and I never want to give up hope for my patients, but I want them to be prepared when death seems inevitable, if not imminent. I raise the subject as a shared concern: "I am concerned that we may be running out of time and may be focusing on things not helping you have the quality of life you want. I am concerned that you might end up in the ER rather than surrounded by your loved ones. I am concerned that not talking about these things, we will be caught unprepared for what is going to happen."

What are the signals that alert you that there is some urgency about the need for that conversation?

Often we start to see that break in a patient's functional status, which typically starts with the patient complaining of being tired all day or dropping ten pounds in a month—markers of frailty. When a patient with advanced cancer consistently needs help with activities of daily living, such as dressing, bathing, and bathroom functions, that's a sign that her body might be shutting down. We also look at serum markers—white blood cell counts, lymphocytes, calcium, and sodium levels in the blood—but the best indication is the patient needing progressively more sleep and progressively more support to get through the day.

continued

What are the main goals of end-of-life care?

Throughout the course of cancer, palliative medicine provides patients with the supportive care they need to control their symptoms and manage their cancer experience. But when patients are approaching the end of their lives, our focus is to ensure that they do not suffer, physically or emotionally. Unfortunately, the symptoms that emerge as a patient is dying are as complex and varied as the patients themselves, but our goal is the same—to minimize discomfort. That also means helping patients and their loved ones plan for the difficult decisions ahead, so that everyone is on the same page and patients' wishes can be honored.

What are the biggest issues confronting patients at the end of their lives?

While many patients remain in denial for a while even after it is clear to doctors and loved ones that the time is near, when they first understand that they are not likely to recover from their cancer, the most common issues are existential ones. "What does it mean to die?" "How will I die?" Patients often assume that a cancer death will be painful and come after a long period of suffering. The first thing I want to do is assure them that this is not going to be the case. That we can control their symptoms. That they will not suffer.

Patients also are fearful that they will die unexpectedly in their sleep. A number of patients come to me with insomnia, and only after talking with them about their wakefulness do we understand that they can't sleep because they are afraid they will die unexpectedly in their sleep. We help them understand that most patients don't die suddenly, but rather, experience progressive sleepiness in the last few weeks of life as their bodies shut down. This gives us time to prepare and to support them through it.

Patients also face a range of worries, including concerns for their families and those around them, such as "Who will take care of my wife, my dog, my farm, my children?" as well as concerns about themselves, such as "Did I do enough, live well enough, take enough care of myself?" Also, it is not unusual for patients to feel angry about their time being cut short. I have had patients as young as fourteen and as old as eighty-four tell me they have been robbed of their due time. Sometimes people feel guilty about the burden they are placing on those around them to provide care; others feel frustrated or experience a loss of purpose—"Why am I still here if I can't do anything or be of any use to anyone?"

Patients face a variety of physical symptoms as well, as their lives come to an end. There are symptoms that relate to the specific type or location of cancer, as well as increasing fatigue and lack of appetite. Usually, patients with advanced cancer succumb to multiorgan failure, which is experienced as progressive sleepiness as the liver and kidneys stop doing their jobs and the brain starts to become "intoxicated" with unreleased toxins (this is called metabolic encephalopathy).

continued

What steps can be taken to deal with the physical issues?

By understanding the type and source of a patient's discomfort, we can prescribe the right type of medication, or even procedure, to ameliorate the pain. Nerve pain can be treated differently than bone pain or pain related to a specific tumor site. Difficulty breathing and anxiety have specific remedies, too, so it starts with understanding what the patient needs in order not to suffer.

How do you help patients achieve emotional readiness for an impending death?

Being emotionally ready for death is a challenge for most patients, as well as for their family members and even their doctors. We all start out fighting cancer, being convinced that we will win in the battle against the disease. It can be very difficult to make the switch to accepting that it wasn't meant to be, to not feel the urge to continue to fight or feel bad that one is "losing" the battle. Even patients who are spiritual and seem to have a personal understanding of death may not be ready to give up the fight. Humans are very good at holding opposing ideas in our minds at the same time, which makes it easy for us to maintain a desire to prolong life even when we know that life may be ending.

To be a good doctor, I have to be sensitive to what my patients are thinking—where they are in their process of acceptance—so that I can guide them and help them make peace with it. I encourage them to say their goodbyes, make the apologies they never quite got to, say the thank-yous they always wish they had, and share their peace and acceptance with their family members. But some patients just can't get there. You can't make people ready if they don't want to talk about it. I let patients know that while I remain hopeful, I never want to see them suffer. If we can start by acknowledging the possibility that things might not work out, we can build on that over time.

What are some of the complicating forces that make management of these issues challenging when a patient is approaching death?

Often there is a readiness discrepancy between the patient and the family. A patient who has been experiencing a physical slowdown and recognizes that death is at hand is more likely to accept it. But many times, I receive a phone call from a member of the patient's family concerned that Mom or Dad is sleeping all the time, and something must be wrong, and can you meet me in the ER? Then I have to reassure the caller, "You have done all that you can, you have taken good care of Mom or Dad, but is this what Mom or Dad would want in the end?"

What can be done to ensure a patient's dignity at the end of her life?

The most important thing is to honor the patient's wishes. Does the patient want life support or does the patient want

continued

to die at home? Would the patient welcome home care? Hospice care? These are conversations that should be had in advance so that those around the patient can support him or her in the best way. It is tricky because as a society, we feel shame in needing others to bathe us, feed us, and care for us at the end of life, and death at home happens less and less frequently, so we no longer know how to support a patient through death at home. Families struggle to accept the death of a loved one and want to rush to the ER, but patients may not want to be on life support when it only prolongs their discomfort.

Palliative care is a quality standard. Every major cancer center is going to have it and it is your right as a patient, or as a patient's loved one, to ask for a palliative-care consult. You don't have to wait until you are burdened with physical symptoms and seeking pain relief; even depression and existential distress and questions about death can be brought to a palliative-care consult. Unfortunately, suffering is an element of advanced cancer, and palliative care can't eliminate all of it, but a doctor can help you glide through the worst of it. A good life incorporates a good death, and asking for palliative care can help.

For more information about palliative care or to find care resources in your community, go to the Center for Palliative Care's Get Palliative Care site at https://getpalliativecare.org.

ADVICE FROM THOSE WHO LEARNED IT THE HARD WAY

Accepting and preparing for end-stage cancer is one of the most challenging ordeals a patient or loving caretaker can face. And whether you are the patient adjusting to the reality that you might not have much life left, or the loving caregiver knowing you are losing the center of your life, the grief of that loss can be overwhelming. Each of us must face that loss and address our fears in a way that is true to our lives. Some will turn to religion and faith, others to practicality and hope. And most will find gradual acceptance of the inevitable.

True to his independence, Jeremy recommended, "Continue to live your life the way you want to, as long as possible. There are folks who will want to tell you how to live, and make decisions for you, but you know what is best for you." Carol agreed. "You know yourself. So you need to deal with it in the way that is best for you, whatever that may be. You have to find your peace and strength. For me, it was family, friends, and going to the woods."

But Paul suggested seeking palliative care early. "Pain and depression are real. You don't want to be caught unprepared for those." And David said, "You've got to be realistic, but that is no reason not to enjoy life. Antidepressants and therapy can help a lot to make the best of the time you have."

Kevin advised that, when caring for a loved one, you straddle the line, making sure you "keep looking for solutions and get the best possible care, but keep the patient comfortable and acknowledge reality." Audrey agreed, and cautioned about the need to remain flexible. "You don't know what you are going to get from day to day, so you have to be ready for anything. And when the grief hits, find a way to get a dose of natural dopamine—take a walk, laugh, surround yourself with people who want you to be happy, and slowly you will find your footing again."

Ann R. advocated allowing others in. "Let your friends help you; don't say no when they offer. You need them to be there for you. And be sure to ask lots of questions. Maybe you don't want to hear the answers, but you need to ask questions to help your patient manage." Maria agreed. "You have to know how to assert yourself when you need something. You can't wait for someone to offer. Being clear with friends about what you or the patient needs makes it easier, although sometimes it's hard to know what that is."

As Randi said after the death of her husband, "It's changed over time for me. I'm not the same and never will be the same. The pain and loss remain, but it doesn't feel as though the bomb just hit. At significant times in life, the feelings get stirred up again. But we're still us. Life is not the same. But, alongside the sadness and yearning, joy has returned to our lives. Cancer cannot destroy love."

8

CUTTING LOOSE: LIFE AFTER TREATMENT AND PHYSICAL RECOVERY

"All changes, even the most longed for, have their melancholy; for what we leave behind us is a part of ourselves."

—Anatole France

For many cancer patients, the end of treatment is the beginning of a whole new ordeal, with physical, emotional, and practical considerations that make life anything but normal. Often we are physically depleted from treatment, with side effects continuing long past the final encounter. Uncertainty about recurrence remains high, and the adrenalin and drive that have carried us through treatment abate, leaving us in a state of suspended animation. We are not yet well, and yet, in theory, no longer sick. We've been cut loose from the watchfulness of regular medical intervention with a cheery "See you in three months," yet told to be vigilant for symptoms and signs of possible recurrence.

Everyone around us, including loved ones and bosses and friends, assumes that we are well and ready to step back into our old lives, when the reality of doing so still seems overwhelming. Nearly 90 percent of patients experience some type of physical concern, 80 percent complain of emotional issues, and almost half have practical challenges.[1] As Melanie said after finishing her breast cancer treatment, "I felt set adrift, sort of like Elsa the lioness [in *Born Free*] being put back into the wild. I had so many lingering questions and concerns."

Physical Residue

Fatigue is one of the most common complaints of patients after the completion of treatment. While we all feel tired from time to time, fatigue interferes with your ability to function. You wake up tired or can't make it through the day without taking a nap. And fatigue can affect job performance, your relationships, even your mood. As Patricia discovered after she and her husband had both made it through treatment, the fatigue is problematic.

> When we were in the midst of crisis, we were so focused on what we had to do. It was a project, and we are both competent people moving through the world with many benefits. But now I'm not as strong as I was, and that creates limitations to how we can think about our future.

Sometimes even the little things can be hard, as Carol discovered after multiple rounds of treatment for recurrent ovarian cancer.

> I used to have more energy and gardened and did everything around the house. Now I'm exhausted, and I know [my energy] is not likely to ever come back. It makes me angry that I can't do simple things anymore. Just carrying a kitchen chair into the bedroom exhausted me. Going up and down stairs, walking, it's all so tiring. I just want my energy back.

In addition to suffering from fatigue, 53 percent of patients are left with some type of limitation on their physical ability due to impairments of the structure or function of their muscles, bones, heart, nerves, or hormones.[2] Some of this deterioration is likely due to the deconditioning that comes with enforced bed rest or the sedentary lifestyle many of us adopt as a result of treatment, but sometimes it's the unintended consequence of the disease or treatment itself. From the extreme impairments of graft-versus-host disease as a result of bone-marrow transplants to the more-common systemic changes from hormone suppression, treatment takes its toll. Pain, neuropathy, muscle damage, lymphedema, and digestive and sexual dysfunction all make transitioning to the next phase that much harder. As Cass explained after she was finished with breast cancer treatment, it can be a snowball effect.

> I was fine throughout treatment, and it was such a relief when they said that I was done. I thought I

would just get on with life. But then I developed a burn from the radiation. My breast was so swollen and sore. So there was new treatment for that. My doctor also prescribed an aromatase inhibitor to suppress estrogen and prevent any additional cancer. That's fine, but it leaches calcium from your bones and so I have developed osteopenia and had two microfractures of my toes just from walking. The medication also causes joint pain and slows the metabolism, so I gained weight. But I couldn't walk because of the fractures in my toes. My oncologist also suggested I take some sort of Fosamax [alendronic acid] for the osteopenia, but I've heard that causes problems too. It just seems that it's never really over.

For Jane T., who had a radical hysterectomy for cervical cancer, the side effects after treatment prevented her from feeling like herself again. "My lymph system went haywire, and I was dripping lymph fluid from my surgical wounds for months. Plus, my doctor removed my cervix and shortened my vagina in the surgery, making sex painful. I am glad to have recovered from cancer, but I wish the doctors were more sensitive to these side issues, which can be almost as challenging as the disease itself."

The likelihood of some type of physical aftereffect can be influenced by other illnesses, genetic sensitivity to treatment, the dose of various treatments received, or even age and general health and fitness, making it hard for doctors to guess in advance who may feel it. But as Bill said after his run-in with lymphoma, "We are all getting older and things go wrong. Having been given a diagnosis of cancer, when something goes wrong, you ask, 'Is it cancer? Was it the treatment? Or is it just age?' It's hard to know."

Practical Considerations

Physical effects can create some real practical considerations as well. It can be hard to return to "normal life" if fatigue prevents you from meeting your responsibilities, you're getting used to a new ostomy bag, you lack the physical strength to lug your groceries into the house, or you discover any number of other limitations. But there can be practical pressures and needs to juggle as well. Jane T. struggled after completing treatment for her cervical cancer.

> I'm self-employed, but I couldn't work for about a month, and didn't know when I could go back to it. I couldn't trust my work when I was on painkillers, but gaps in my insurance coverage meant a significant need for cash. It costs gazillions to have cancer and a hysterectomy! The insurance process itself was stressful, and the hospital bills were incomprehensible—what's covered, what isn't, what was deducted or not deducted? I had to ease back into work in order to get some cash flow, but I'm not sure I was at my best for a while.

Crystal started easing back to work three weeks after her mastectomy because she felt she had to be ready to attend a professional conference that was scheduled for five weeks after surgery.

I was exhausted. I had to take naps every day. I started with about an hour a day and then built up from there. If you checked in with my friends, they would have said I seemed normal, but I used to be a high-energy person, and found I had to take it slow.

At the airport on my way to the conference, they gave me a pat-down because I was wearing a headscarf. [The] TSA [Transportation Security Administration] was not at all sympathetic. And the airline attendants don't understand and aren't helpful either. There was no way I could put my suitcase overhead. I had to change the way I travel, and even booked a wheelchair so I didn't have to carry or lift anything.

Param, whose leukemia was medically managed for a number of years, had a bone-marrow transplant when his disease progressed. Balancing his health needs against those of his work and family was a challenge.

My girls were eleven and nine years old when I had the transplant, and explaining to them what was going on was so hard. They stayed with their grandparents while I was hospitalized, but my elder daughter thought she had to run the family, had to be the adult in the household while her mom and I were away. I was the focus of attention, and the children felt it. It was hard for them, but we couldn't get back to normal any faster than we did.

Home responsibilities can be especially difficult if you are a single parent. Stephanie had three young kids at home and had to get back to work to support them pretty quickly after her breast cancer surgery and chemo. But as a hospital nurse, she found it complicated.

> I didn't want my patients to know I had been sick and wanted to look as uniformly healthy as possible. Mostly I managed to get away with it. But I had one patient who went through chemo at the same time I did. That was more than a little awkward.

Emotional Challenges

These lingering physical issues, side effects, and practical stressors contribute to what would be an emotionally charged time with or without them. Many patients feel conflicted at the end of treatment, not sure how to re-center their lives in the absence of ongoing medical intervention. As Melanie said, "I was depressed, and I didn't understand why I was so sad. But I had this sense that I was wandering in the desert, not sure where I was going next. And in a fit of emotional meltdown, I walked away from my own business. I could no longer do what I had always done."

While not everyone makes life-altering decisions in the weeks following the end of treatment, depression and disorientation are not uncommon. Eliot frequently found himself in tears after he had completed immunotherapy for metastatic melanoma.

I had been up for so many months, and physically never felt ill before diagnosis or during treatment, so it was hard to comprehend that I had cancer. It was only afterward that I could relax, once it was behind me and the enormity of it washed over me. Then I was so tearful. I'm good at managing my way through intense projects, but it's when the pressure is off that you can reflect and take in what just happened.

Part of the emotional response is the retreat from high alert that propels one through the experience, but often the anxiety about recurrence remains. Patricia found this continued vigilance particularly challenging.

It was hard. Henry felt it more than I did, and it was hard for him to talk about the many unknowns that were left. We were living with a sense of uncertainty. We didn't know what life would bring, but the cancer was at hand at all times. We were on alert and it was really lonely at times. We didn't want all our interaction with others to be about health and didn't want his business to be jeopardized by the potential threat of cancer returning. So we held it all in.

Lingering anxiety can take its toll, not just immediately after the completion of treatment but for months to come as we continue to bounce back from the experience and worry about the future. Loretta noticed that she wasn't herself six months after finishing treatment for breast cancer.

I was sitting in this place of remembering what had happened and what was going on and found that I was depressed. I didn't want to do things—I wasn't myself. My doctor suggested I get some therapy and sent me to a cancer psychologist. The first day, I walked in, sat down, looked at the therapist, and just started sobbing for a long time. When the therapist asked me what I was feeling, I said that I had been holding on to my strength for the past several months, being strong about what's going on, and I just can't be strong anymore. "That's a very normal experience," she said. "A lot of people are strong and then can't hold on anymore." So I just let go of it there and then. It was a delayed reaction of complete and total letting go.

The psychologist knew how to help me, to allow me to have these feelings, and not feel as though there was something wrong with me. She assured me that this was a normal reaction to a life-threatening experience. Even though I had extremely good results, it didn't diminish my feelings, didn't mean that I didn't have a right to feel bad. I was feeling guilty about feeling sorry for myself, but she said it was okay. That allowed me to work through my emotions and come to the point after about six weeks where I could acknowledge that I had had cancer, that I wasn't going through this alone, and I was lucky to be a survivor.

It is also not uncommon to have self-identity issues after a life- and body-altering event such as cancer. And while some of the disfigurement may be temporary or externally concealed, often the psychological impact lingers long after the physical changes are no longer evident. Jeremy found that the multiple surgeries and treatments for his rare cancer of the appendix necessitated redefining himself after a lifetime of physical strength and ability.

> I was the alpha, at least in my own mind. I had a competitiveness that told me, "I can beat you at this, can outrun you, can crawl farther than you." I used to do push-ups with my kids on my back or bench-press them until they were fifteen and twelve. I took being fit very seriously and would run, bike, lift weights, go trail hiking, etc. [Now] there's a huge discrepancy between who I think I am and who I really am, and it's very isolating.

Jill R. was struck by the lingering emotional toll from the disfigurement of cancer after her double mastectomy and chemotherapy.

> Along the way, my mom asked why I would bother with the reconstruction, but when your breasts are there, it's easy not to worry about them. I didn't want to have an abnormal body. I had drains from the mastectomy for months, which I carried in my suit jacket to work. I used to worry that if I pulled out a pen, it might be a drain instead.
>
> My husband didn't think it should matter and tried to make me feel as loved and desired as before, that my breasts were not important to him. But it does matter. Just having a body that is not the healthy, whole body that you were—it's a problem.

SCIENCE SIDEBAR: THE SCIENCE OF RECOVERY

So what exactly is happening in there that prevents us from jumping right back into life the day after treatment ends? There are several interrelated drivers of our need for some recovery time, including continued healing from the assaults of treatment, ongoing imbalances of metabolism, hormones, and cytokines, and general deconditioning. In addition, the psychological impact of these lingering issues keeps most folks in a state of ongoing stress, further exacerbating the symptoms.

Under the best circumstances, physical healing takes time. The evidence of a simple cut on the finger may disappear within a couple of weeks, but the average surgical scar is not considered fully healed for six months to a year.[3] It takes that long for the body to make the right kind of cells, bring them to the right place, grow the appropriate vascular structure to support them, and remove and reprocess unnecessary scar tissue.

Similarly, chemotherapy and radiation cause side effects that take time to heal. Although both treatments target rapidly dividing cancer cells, other cells that have a high rate of turnover, such as skin and mucus membranes, can be damaged too, increasing the need for healing and adding time to the recovery process. Radiation also has the potential to change the structure of skin and connective tissue in the area surrounding the target, and can affect the vascular structure of the tissue as well, giving the body still more repair work to do.[4]

One of the tricks the body uses to prevent the spread of

continued

cancer is cellular senescence—essentially aging the cells and shutting down their ability to replicate. Senescence also plays a role in wound healing, preventing scar tissue from growing out of control. But cellular stress, including the stress of radiation and chemotherapy, can trigger excess senescence. And unfortunately, one of the side effects of cellular senescence is inflammation,[5] meaning that more pro-inflammatory cytokines are released, which further increases fatigue. It can take months for the body to clear the excess senescent cells and for inflammatory markers to return to normal.

LIQUID DAMAGES

In addition to damaging tissue, treatment also attacks our fast-replicating blood cells, including platelets, red blood cells, and white blood cells. Platelets, which play an important role in tissue repair and regeneration,[6] are killed off by chemotherapy and radiation—just when we need them most, they've gone missing. While we make billions of them every day, they have a life span of only ten to twelve days, so it can be tough on the body to play catch-up, which often results in bone pain as the marrow goes into overdrive.

Similarly, red blood cell counts can drop significantly, leading to decreases in circulating hemoglobin and an inability to provide sufficient oxygen to our muscles. More fatigue. Although doctors may postpone treatment for a week or more if blood cell counts dip too low, it's not unusual to end treatment with a deficit of up to one-third of our usual healthy counts. We generate about 2.4 million new red blood cells every second, but that's a small fraction of the 10 trillion or so we may have lost. Given that red blood cells last only for three to four months, there is constant turnover, but it can be hard to build back the lost cells while maintaining daily turnover rates.

The immune system also takes a hit thanks to a significant die-off of white blood cells. (Treatment to suppress the immune system is one of the things doctors count on when preparing patients for stem-cell or bone-marrow transplants.) Since the immune system is the body's actual mechanism for initiating homeostasis,[7] it's no surprise that when it's not functioning at peak capacity, it can take time for metabolism and hormone balance and even circadian rhythms to reestablish norms after cancer and its treatment.

One cytokine produced by the immune system, transforming growth factor-b (TGF-b), helps regulate cell activity, including signaling when cells should grow, migrate, die, develop a blood supply, and do everything else we count on them to do.[8] But TGF-b can promote increased inflammation rather than turning it down, further prolonging the imbalance and fatigue, and slowing the regeneration of cells necessary for healing. Meanwhile, those dreaded pro-inflammatory cytokines (see the Science Sidebar in chapter 3), so essential to healing but with the potential to drive sickness behavior and depression, are still working in overdrive.[9] No wonder we don't bounce back.

THE DOWNWARD SPIRAL

Unfortunately, these deficits gang up on us to make the recovery process a slow, uphill battle. Even if we didn't turn

continued

into total couch potatoes, there would be some deconditioning that happens due to the side effects of treatment. It's highly likely that we suffered some—if not many—days of not feeling fully ourselves. As a result, there's a good chance we didn't maintain the level of activity we were used to before the diagnosis, whatever that baseline may have been, and so don't end treatment with the level of robustness we previously thought of as "normal." For most of us, the whole treatment period is a slow downward slope of deconditioning. No matter how determined we are to keep moving, we end up being a little—or a lot—weaker than we were at the beginning. Decreases in hemoglobin mean we have less energy and are less likely to feel like going for a walk, much less head to the gym, so we get progressively weaker. We give ourselves license to skip the walk, friends bring dinner (obviating the need for us to shop and cook), and we spend more time sitting and napping.

Studies have shown that in just twenty days of continuous bed rest, even young, healthy men lose 27 percent of their aerobic fitness, equivalent to aging thirty years.[10] And reconditioning takes time. We need to rebuild hemoglobin levels, rebuild muscle strength, and rebuild the nutritional inputs that fuel muscles, which often are depleted during days of languid queasiness.[11]

Human bodies work hard all the time to maintain a balanced metabolic rate. But with stress and illness, metabolic demand can increase as much as 40 percent, even if we are not exercising. At the same time, after months of altered appetite, we may not be achieving the same nutritional balance we had before. If we are at all malnourished at the time we are trying to heal, or are further stressed by infection or injury, organs may go into overdrive, borrowing protein and other nutrients from skin and muscles in order to function, contributing to weakness.[12]

In addition, cancer and its treatment can result in disruptions to the endocrine system, meaning hormones are released at the wrong levels and at the wrong times of day, upsetting circadian rhythms, sleeping habits, and neuromuscular function. We are likely to experience these disturbances as difficulty sleeping, muscle aches and pains, cognitive impairment, and, yes, more fatigue.[13]

ALL IN THE HEAD

These physical challenges take their toll on us emotionally too. Unfortunately, lack of physical activity can contribute to depression. In one study, physically inactive individuals were 45 percent more likely to be depressed than active ones. And there is a similar link between inactivity and anxiety.[14] In addition to being less physically active, many of us tend to hibernate during cancer, limiting our social activity. And yet for most people, a decrease in social activity also can contribute to the stress reaction and depression, further heightening discomfort. While the systemic imbalances are physical, we experience those imbalances in our minds, making it hard to reverse the pattern.

For some of us, a couple of sunny days or a shared laugh or a well-timed hug is enough to start the upward climb toward

continued

physical and emotional recovery. But for others, the symbolic bell ringing at the end of chemo just isn't going to do it. Many patients find they need antidepressants, stimulants, pain medication, counseling, and other kinds of support to get them out of their treatment funk, and just about all of us will need the one thing we never have enough of—time.

Eventually, we heal. Systems stabilize, and the body returns to homeostasis, maybe not the same as before cancer, but enough so that we begin to feel more normal. We still have constant reminders of the ordeal we have survived—scars, funky hair, perhaps an ongoing maintenance therapy or hormone-suppressing medication, and frequent medical check-ins—but we can begin to put the experience behind us. As Crystal said, "I realized one morning that it was no longer painful just to get out of bed. That was when I could finally stop thinking about cancer every day."

SIDEBAR: Q AND A ON THE IMPORTANCE OF EXERCISE

Martha Eddy, EdD in movement science, is an **exercise physiologist and somatic therapist** with more than twenty-five years of research and practice in the field of enhancing wellness through movement. As the **founding director of Moving for Life**, a dance and exercise program dedicated to helping older adults and people of all ages challenged by cancer, she works with cancer patients in all stages of their recovery using research-supported methods to improve their physical and emotional well-being.

What role does exercise play in recovery from and management of cancer?

Exercise is an integral part of treatment and should be part of a comprehensive recovery plan. Many leading hospitals and cancer centers offer exercise programs for their patients as part of cancer treatment. Exercise has been shown to create real physiological changes that aid in recovery by counteracting some of the deleterious effects of treatment and improving the management of symptoms. Aerobic exercise in particular helps detoxify and strengthen the body at the cellular level, allowing patients to get back to feeling healthy sooner.

How does exercise help the physical recovery process?

A properly structured exercise program can help increase mobility and range of motion, decrease the likelihood and severity of lymphedema, increase energy to combat fatigue, and reduce symptoms of neuropathy and joint pain. Exercise also helps with weight management (which is frequently an issue during treatment), leading to indirect changes that buttress against cancer.

Most importantly, exercise has been shown to reduce the recurrence of cancer. Increasing evidence suggests that exercise, particularly aerobic exercise, creates biologic and metabolic changes that protect against cancer. It also stimulates changes in the way our genes behave as they reproduce, affecting DNA repair and the aging process. Exercise also stimulates the immune system, reduces inflammation and oxidative stress (the burden on our bodies from using oxygen in the air we breathe to metabolize food into energy—the natural "rusting" that ages us from the inside out), and even speeds digestion time, which reduces the risk of colon cancer.[15]

How does exercise affect brain chemistry and emotions?

Exercise has been shown to have many benefits to how we think and feel, including reduced fatigue, depression, anxiety, and stress, as well as increased joy and improved body image. Many of these benefits are thought to come about because of the release of endorphins and monoamines when we exercise, but the distraction of a healthy escape and an increase in core body temperature are also thought to contribute to improved mood, along with exposure to sunlight when exercising out of doors.

When we exercise at the right level of exertion, we kick-start the exertion/recuperation cycle, changing the status of the autonomic nervous system, which helps lower both sympathetic nervous system activity (the fight/flight/freeze mechanisms) and our perception of stress. This is an important part of the healing process and has a dramatic effect on the brain.

However, in order to derive the mood-enhancing benefits of exercise, you have to enjoy it, not perceive it as a chore. If we force ourselves to do exercise we hate or are critical of ourselves for not performing well enough, we tend not to benefit as greatly from the effort. The key to gaining the most from exercise is to find something that is pleasurable so as to get the endorphin rush. Besides, success breeds success, making it more likely that you will incorporate it into your life, making it a habit that persists long after you recover.

What research has been done to support the use of exercise to improve body and mind after cancer?

A number of studies have shown that cancer patients who exercise have 30 to 60 percent lower rates of recurrence and improved survival rates compared to sedentary patients.[16] Most of the research has been done with breast, colorectal, and prostate cancer patients, and most studies show a correlation, not causation. However, there is growing evidence to suggest that exercise itself is the cause of reduced cancer rates in some types of cancer. Studies have also shown that

continued

exercise enhances the quality of life of cancer patients by decreasing fatigue, perception of pain, sleep disturbances, anxiety, and depression while helping patients lose weight and contributing to emotional well-being by improving body image, self-esteem, sexuality, and social functioning. This is particularly important in estrogen-based cancers because the loss of fat helps reduce the chance of recurrence. Muscle strength also increases the pull on the bones and can be an antidote to developing osteopenia and osteoporosis, common side effects of hormone-suppression medication.

At what point in treatment/recovery is it best to start exercising?

Most patients can start exercising four to six weeks after surgery (once cleared by their doctors) and can exercise throughout treatment, but it depends on how healthy and active you were before your illness. Those who were fit and active before diagnosis are more likely to feel comfortable exercising sooner, but treatment is exhausting, so they may need to work at a slower pace than before their disease. This requires patience but is worth it. You'll stick with it longer when it feels good. Patients who were not active before, or who are older or overweight, may need a longer time to ramp up to regular exercise. Starting with seated exercise can be a good option.

Everyone can benefit from exercise, but how long it takes until people feel the benefits will also vary with exercise experience. Some people bounce back quickly; others need more time before they start to see the benefits of their hard work. Taking naps and rests is an important part of both treatment recovery and post-workout resiliency. Schedule your exercise wisely.

What type of exercise helps patients with cancer? Does it matter what type of exercise one does?

The surprise from our research in the 1990s was that aerobic exercise is key. Swimming, dancing, hiking, even walking—anything that increases blood flow and raises your heart rate—are beneficial. A program that includes a warm-up, some aerobic activity, gentle stretching and strengthening, and a cool-down period is the best way to get started if you have been inactive. Aerobic training reduces fatigue by teaching the body to get the most energy out of ingested nutrients. It also encourages the production of red blood cells, which can be destroyed by chemotherapy and inactivity, and increases blood flow, which brings oxygen to all the cells, including those in your brain. This increased blood flow is important to help with wound healing and the reduction of joint pain, neuropathy, and lymphedema, and has the added benefit of helping prevent heart disease.

Yoga has been adapted for cancer patients for decades and is great for stress reduction and flexibility; if someone is deconditioned or doing a more rigorous yoga class it may even become aerobic. Exercises that require movement and stretching help increase flexibility and range of motion by easing the body into new positions, but it's important always to avoid pain, working within your own range and gradually adding more. In order to prevent muscle strain and

continued

reduce scar-tissue damage, it is essential to warm up with some aerobic activity before doing any range-of-motion or stretching exercises or any strength-building exercises. And a final cooldown helps prevent the buildup of lactic acid in the muscles and joints that were active during exercise.

There are also special considerations in structuring an individual exercise plan. To address concerns about lymphedema, exercise that pumps the arms (such as squeezing the fists) and the legs (pushing hard off the foot when walking)—peripheral muscular pumping—can help prevent or minimize the impact of lymphedema, stimulating the flow of lymph fluid back to the heart, where it can be reabsorbed. If neuropathy is an issue, exercises that use pressure to override the pain sensors can reduce pain and may stimulate healthy sensation and (together with increased blood flow) encourage nerve regeneration. And for joint pain, the key is to minimize oxidative stress (which can increase inflammation and pain) by working within a smaller range of motion, taking it slowly and building toward full activity. Losing any extra weight can also help reduce pressure on the joints, and in turn, joint pain.

The key is to listen to your body. If you exercise one day and it wipes you out, maybe take a day off and rest, then try again without pushing it quite so hard. You have to pay attention and adjust. If there is pain, back off. If you are dizzy, don't do anything that will risk a fall—instead, consider seated exercise. If nausea is a problem, avoid fast rotations, bending over, or standing up too quickly. There are lots of ways to adapt an exercise to your individual needs. Be sensible—if your knee hurts, don't jog. It's important to find exercise you enjoy from the beginning so there is a desire to continue. An introvert might prefer working alone, while an extrovert often will benefit from the social, as well as the physical, experience of an exercise class

How much exercise should a patient do?

Most people can benefit from thirty to sixty minutes of exercise, two or three times a week. But that is a goal, not a starting point. If you haven't been active, it's best to start with twelve to fifteen minutes of aerobic activity—even if it's just walking or swaying to music. You want to continue moving throughout your recovery in order to avoid losing healthy skills and developing new symptoms from not moving. Gradually build up to the 150 minutes of exercise a week recommended by the American Cancer Society. This can be thirty minutes of gentle walking five days a week, or anything else that keeps you moving. But be sure you make it fun, because keeping at it is what counts!

ADVICE FROM THOSE WHO LEARNED IT THE HARD WAY

Physical recovery takes time. It's a slow process that we chip away at over days, weeks, and months. But there are things you can do to help. Patients have found that easing back into work and social life, with proper focus on exercise and ongoing support, all the while taking care of yourself, can speed the process. But, as Catherine said after her mastectomy, "You have to be patient, though, because it took me about eighteen months to get back to normal."

Keeping yourself busy is both a distraction and a good counterweight to the lingering side effects of cancer. As Patricia said, "It's really hard not to let cancer take over, but by focusing on the rest of life, it helps keep things in balance." And if that source of distraction can involve a little physical activity, all the better. Sue M. went back to running as soon as she could. "It was hard to get started again, but gave me such a sense of accomplishment, and a little positive energy," she said. "I highly recommend it."

Many patients retreat from social activity during treatment and aren't quite ready to jump back in when it's over. But there are benefits to having people around. "Cancer is isolating, but reach out, even if it's an online support group. It helps to know you are not going through it alone," said Jeremy. Param agreed. "When you withdraw, that is the challenge. Everyone needs some support, even adjusting after cancer."

While being patient, it helps to take good care of yourself. Christina found meditation, diet, and surrounding herself with positive energy were all helpful as she recovered from esophageal cancer on the heels of breast cancer treatment. "Self-care is so important, especially when you have young kids you worry about," she said. "If you don't take care of yourself, you can't be there to take care of them."

Many patients feel as though they have asked for so much during the treatment phase of the cancer ordeal that it's time to stop asking now that treatment is done. But sometimes it helps to keep asking. "Tell your friends what support you need from them, even after you're done with treatment," said Cass. "I wish I had asked for more, because I know my friends would have been there for me, even though they were as ready for me to be done with cancer as I was." Stephanie agreed. "Let people know what you need. They're happy to keep helping, but don't make them guess," she said.

And if it all feels too overwhelming, ask for professional help as well. As Loretta said, "Don't sit in that place of despair. You have to keep going. Listen to your body, because you know things, and then get the help you need." Crystal agreed. "See a therapist to help you with the emotional upheaval," she said. "It's a life-changing illness and it helps to have the support of a professional along with your friends and family."

Or as Melanie put it, "Some of us pray, some quit working, some reach out, others don't. There's no right way or wrong way, so long as you don't give up and become a walking pity party."

THE NEW NORMAL: WHEN IT'S SAFE TO RESUME LIFE

I can be changed by what
happens to me. But I refuse to
be reduced by it.

—*Maya Angelou*

At some point, we move on. We heal, physically and emotionally, and resume our lives. Some of us quietly slip back into our old lives, barely registering a ripple; some of us are aware of changes in perspective and values as we return to our old lives; and some of us structure entirely new lives, like a phoenix rising from the ashes. Regardless of how life may have outwardly changed, 50 to 80 percent of people with a history of cancer report some added value in their lives as a result of their cancer experiences.[1] These benefits range from strengthened interpersonal relationships to improved clarity of and commitment to life priorities, increased attention to health, renewed spirituality, a feeling of personal strength, and appreciation for one's health, family, friends, and a life no longer taken for granted.[2]

While scientists don't fully understand the drivers behind who feels the greatest impact and why, it appears that the strength of the perceived threat and magnitude of the disruption cancer caused influences the reaction, and the more actively one has focused on coping, the more likely one is to feel some growth or benefit from the experience. It also seems to help if you had social support while coping with your ordeal.[3]

No Grand Promises

Just as we experience cancer in different ways, so too we experience moving on in a variety of ways. For some, the urge is to just put the past aside and get back to life. Steve, who had survived testicular cancer in his thirties, felt less threatened by colon cancer in his fifties and wasn't making any promises about a new life as he wrapped up treatment.

> I remember distinctly, after finishing treatment and CT scans every six months for my first cancer, making so many proclamations. I was going to have this new life and do things differently. Well, that lasted a very short time and then I went back to who I was. The greater the time gap, the more I ignored those proclamations. So now, I don't anticipate being a different person. I'm not making any proclamations. I'm not going to fool myself—I'm just going to go back to living my life the same as I always have.

Sue, who had anticipated a cancer diagnosis for decades before its arrival, also didn't acknowledge any fundamental changes after completing her treatment, but she did feel a greater awareness of how lucky she was in life.

> It was an amazing episode that made me so grateful for the progress of health care, and the support of friends and community. It was astonishing to experience such overt kindness. I am typically reserved about myself and expect that I should take care of myself. But by sharing my bad news with friends, my life was extraordinarily enriched. And it opened my eyes to what others might be going through; it helped me be more aware of other people's needs. I won't say that having cancer changed me, but it gave me a chance to recall who I am and become more so.

For others, graduating from being a cancer patient to being someone with a history of cancer brings clarity to priorities that help focus life. Like Sue, Julie felt enormous gratitude as she reflected on her breast cancer ordeal fifteen years earlier. But she acknowledged a greater shift in her life as a result.

> I felt a heightened sense of awareness, brought on by the illness. I came out of the experience a different person, an emotionally mature person. Cancer also gave me a changed perspective on "ambition." It's not that I'm not ambitious anymore, but I'm no longer envious of other people's successes, and more interested in creating my own vision of success.

I realized with cancer that we have no control over anything—despite what we might like to think. Maybe I can do my laundry with control. Maybe. But there is this whole flexibility of ego that happens when you realize you're not really the one driving the bus. When you understand that you can only "take charge," not take control, it really informs the whole "ambition" thing.

Similarly, Elyse found that cancer helped her focus on her priorities after she recovered from lymphoma.

I feel that clarity of what's important, who I want to spend time with, how I want to spend my life. I came to recognize that I carry around a lot of stress. Cancer pushed me toward realizing that my health has to come first. It also opened the door and allowed me to pivot and explore all sorts of healing for mind, body, and spirit. Most importantly, cancer gave me the opportunity to be present.

That sense of being present and awake to the passing of time, the importance of enjoying life, is a common theme. As Aparna said, looking back on her run-in with breast cancer:

Cancer is a distant memory for me most of the time but it's a milestone in my life because it helped me redefine and reevaluate my life, my goals, attitudes, perspectives. I'm full of gratitude for the lessons my disease taught me, and my attitude toward life has changed. I try to live in the moment and don't postpone my joys. I don't plan too much into the future because I truly believe that if today is well-lived, tomorrow will take care of itself.

At some point, I had an epiphany that the cancer was going to change things for the better. I didn't know how, but I was sure that something good would emerge. The realization was instant, but the change has been gradual, giving me faith in the universe as an abundant, generous, and forgiving entity. I became a more positively spiritual person who learned to choose consciously, take responsibility, lose the victim mindset, and live in the present. Cancer taught me a new way of living. For that, I am and will remain eternally grateful.

Sometimes recovery happens in surprising ways. Shilpi was always an optimist and was sure she would be fine through her breast cancer ordeal, but it left an impression.

When the cancer had been behind me for a couple of years, I was convinced I would never date again, but then I saw someone at a party that I had known for a long time. We hooked up and it healed me in a way. It was never going to be a permanent relationship, but he made it clear that my scar didn't matter to him, and he was comfortable and open to talking about my experience. If I had gone through that process with someone I had just met, it would have been harder. Instead, it was very reaffirming and got me out of the mindset that I was never going to date again.

But I still think about my cancer every day. It is so much a part of me that there isn't any moment of my life that isn't colored by it. On the best days, I feel very lucky that I survived, and on bad days, I can still remind myself that however bad it is, it's not as bad as cancer.

Life-Altering Experience

Other people with a history of cancer find the experience so powerful that they literally change their lives—their personalities, their jobs, even their spouses. Rachel, who had a frightening experience with a deep melanoma on her buttocks, credits that existential crisis with helping her change her life for the better.

I had this really strange experience. All these doctors and total strangers were touching and pinching me to deal with my cancer. But some examined me in gentle, tender, and respectful ways, and one time, I fell to pieces. I know they felt I was crying because I was so scared, which I was. But also, I missed physical intimacy and realized that I had been dying a little bit over the years with the lack of connection with my husband. Cancer brought it to the surface. It gave me clarity—all the usual clutter and distraction fell away. What was left was a kind of pure certainty of what was important and the importance of living to do those things.

We are still co-parenting our children, but it became clear to me that I couldn't waste any more time. I needed to be free of that relationship. It's been a challenging year. I also felt an urgency to say "I love you" to the people in my life that I really cared about. Everything deepened: the way I felt with my kids, my family, my friends. The sense of clarity has faded a bit with time, but it's still there, and I try to act on it every day.

Param found a new sense of fulfillment by getting involved in an advocacy organization and helping others deal with cancer after his bone-marrow transplant for leukemia.

I feel blessed to have had chronic myelogenous leukemia. Thanks to The Max Foundation, I was able to get the medicine I needed and have a good quality of life, so I feel inspired to advocate for others. I have become a hard-core volunteer with The Max Foundation. I am a very positive person, and I can create positive energy for others living with cancer. It's interesting because my career really accelerated after my diagnosis, and I think it was because I became a stronger person—more focused and less fearful. It is hard to be mindful when you are afraid.

Jennifer echoed that sentiment after recovering from her third recurrence of ovarian cancer and launching a ministry to support cancer patients and others in need at home and in Africa.

Cancer helped me to see exactly who I was supposed to be. I will never be sad that I had cancer. God has shown me exactly what my direction is, what I am supposed to do with my life. I have always been devoted to God and involved in my church. But after cancer, I felt that I was standing on the edge, looking out over this beautiful valley, and I had to go through this incredibly deep journey of faith to get to the other side. This is where God wants me to be. Now I am 10 million percent deeper into my faith than ever before.

Nina, who declared that she "had cancer for about two weeks," was so motivated to help others by her brief experience with ovarian and endometrial cancer that she launched an international aid organization to provide support to patients with cancer in developing countries.

I used to be a photographer. But after cancer, I felt compelled to help, because I knew how fortunate I was that I got off so easy. I began searching for an idea and set out to make a photo documentary to show the universality of cancer. But once I truly saw the need, I had to jump in and help. Cancer gave me the opportunity to change my life. Now I feel empowered, fearless to try or do anything. What's the worst that could happen? Cancer highlights how important it is to do something meaningful with your life.

Terri expressed a similar sense that cancer and a badly timed breakup had given her a chance to really shake things up. After recovering from a double mastectomy when she was in her thirties, she founded A Fresh Chapter, a volunteer corps of cancer patients, survivors, and caregivers focused on healing by helping others.

> I've always been type A, locked in the illusion that I can control everything. So I was very shocked to have cancer. It was not part of the plan. But it was an opportunity for me to create a secondary character, to become someone who was braver than before, and take ownership of the negative experience.
>
> When I was done with treatment, I planned a trip to do some volunteer work in a part of the world I had never visited. I got on the plane feeling, "Poor me, I had cancer." But when I got off the plane in South Africa, my perspective started to shift. There was a two-year-old boy who I worked with who had such a profound impact on me. He didn't care that I'd had cancer. New people I met didn't care who I had been before. It gave me the luxury of asking "Who do I want to be now?"
>
> I met women who struggled to feed and clothe kids; I saw the aftermath of apartheid and unspeakable atrocities. I realized that even though I had been through cancer, I wasn't alone in struggling. Everybody struggles. People go through so much and find resilience. Who am I to feel sorry for myself? Given the opportunities that I have, who am I to stay in this place of feeling like a victim? It gave me a sense of empowerment, but also of responsibility. I felt I couldn't waste it.
>
> There is this notion that cancer is supposed to make us great and that we are all supposed to go off

and do amazing things and change the world. That is way too much pressure. But what really motivated me was I was just so disappointed in where my life was after cancer. I had been through so much treatment. I had thought my relationship was strong, and that since we had made it through cancer, we could make it through anything. And I knew I didn't want to go back to my old job. I could sit there and be angry about what wasn't possible, the many things I couldn't control, or I could figure out what was possible. And what started as something that would light me up turned into something bigger.

Not everyone needs to change the world, or even a small part of it, after coming through a cancer experience. But most of us want to reflect on it and incorporate whatever it is we learned about ourselves and others into life as we move forward. As Anne said after recovering from her third round of ovarian cancer, "Your individual 'well again' is up to you; it's not just medical, spiritual, or having a good time, but it's opening yourself with joy to the adventure that you are on, and believing that this will deepen the effect you make in the world and vice versa." True healing is about personal growth, whatever that means to you.

SCIENCE SIDEBAR: EMOTIONAL RECOVERY AND RESILIENCY

Emotional recovery takes place in the brain. And since each of us is wired differently, influenced by our genetics, past experiences, and particular course with the disease, that's going to mean a unique starting place and recovery path for each of us. But regardless of where we begin, the brain needs to learn to deal with the threat of cancer. Like soldiers recovering from PTSD, we slowly teach the brain not to jump at the sound of every scary noise, turning down the automatic stress reaction that drives fear, leads to anxiety and depression, contributes to fatigue, and makes the whole cancer experience such an emotionally volatile time.

There are two important concepts that underlie emotional recovery. The first is what neuroscientists refer to as neuroplasticity—essentially the idea that the brain is constantly changing and rewiring itself.[4] That rewiring is more effective when we are young—just watch a child pick up a new language or sport versus an adult struggling with the same tasks. But developing new connections in the brain happens every day. It's what allows us to form memories, learn to use the latest technology, and even walk with achy knees.

At the same time, it is helpful to remember the stress response that we first encountered in chapter 1. When something triggers fear, the automatic part of the nervous system kicks into gear. The hypothalamus initiates a chain reaction that results in the release of stress hormones that put us into fight-or-flight mode. And while the hypothalamus, pituitary

continued

gland, and adrenal cortex play a key role in responding to stress, resilience and the process of coping with stress are much more complex. Scientists now think that several parts of the brain, the immune system, and even the gut microbiome contribute to resilience.[5] Given the involvement of the immune system, it's no surprise that it can take a while for us to regain emotional health. As we saw in chapter 8, the body—including the immune system—can take months, even years, to reestablish homeostasis.

Most of what we know about changes in the body and brain that lead to resilience comes from studies with mice, but the unfortunate experience of numerous war veterans returning with PTSD has taught us a lot about how to apply that knowledge to stress recovery. One of the most-effective treatments for trauma is "stress inoculation," which trains the brain not to go into overdrive any time it encounters a stressful situation by building new neural circuits that suppress amygdala activity. And every day that we live with our cancer diagnosis, every day that we make it through treatment, every time we get good news on scans and tests is like a stress inoculation that trains the brain not to panic about cancer. While some of this repatterning seems to occur on its own, the more active we are in helping ourselves cope, the faster this process happens, with more neurocircuits developing and relief happening in a shorter period of time.[6]

Those who struggle with what scientists refer to as a "failure of plasticity,"[7] which makes it hard for the brain to rewire after stress, are often stuck with fear, anxiety, depression, and other symptoms. Experience with PTSD patients suggests that cognitive-behavioral therapy, controlled-exposure therapy, and cognitive-processing therapy, sometimes coupled with antidepressant and anti-inflammatory medication, are most helpful in building a strongly rewired network,[8] and would be beneficial for cancer patients as well. The science of emotional resilience is still new, but it's worth reaching out for help if months go by without relief.

ADVICE FROM THOSE WHO LEARNED IT THE HARD WAY

Many patients are surprised to discover how resilient they are when they finally see cancer in the rearview mirror. Things just start to feel normal again, whatever that might be, and life goes on. As Shilpi said, "It is amazing how much our bodies can take, and then you are better." But if you're still wondering how to put it all in perspective, those who have been there suggest a few measures that might be sound advice for life in general.

Without meaning to sound like a sneaker commercial, Mary G. advocated for actively embracing life. "Just do it," she said. "There is much you had to put aside while putting your life on hold, but now you can make up for lost time." Or, as Deborah put it, "Live every day to the max, but save for the future too, so that you learn from yesterday, make use of today, and plan for the future."

Others recommend trying to gain some perspective on the ordeal. As Bob said, "I think it helps to look at the cancer experience as a gift in a strange package. It helps us grow and be a better person to the world around us." Aparna echoed that sentiment. "Cancer taught me a new way of living," she said. "It helps if you can find a way to feel gratitude, despite what you've been through."

Noreen found that she was suddenly aware of cancer everywhere, and that awareness could be beneficial. "Once you understand how many lives it really does touch, you can use that knowledge to change how you interact," she said. "Look at the people around you and assume that some are going through challenges as you did. It makes you see people differently." Anne agreed. "Survivorship is fellowship," she said. "There are so many of us out there who have been or are or will be going through this. It can help if you keep this in mind."

But it's important not to judge yourself or others in the process. Michelle said, "It's okay to slip back into bad habits and resume the life you had. Cancer doesn't have to be life-changing." Carl weighed in with a similar sentiment. "There are a lot of articles and books out there on the gifts of cancer," he said. "But it's not for everyone. You don't have to reinvent yourself because you survived a disease."

Sooner or later, the experience begins to fade. "At some point you realize, it's just not in your head anymore," Nancy H. said. "It's okay to just forget about it." Urvi agreed. "It is easy to forget the unpleasant things in life," she said. "So just let it go."

With resilience, we get back to living. And, like a helium balloon released from the finish line of a long race, once let go, the big ordeal fades away, in time becoming not such a big ordeal after all.

RESOURCES

General Cancer Information and Support

- **American Cancer Society (cancer.org)**
  Cancer information, answers, and hope.

- **CancerCare (cancercare.org)**
  Counseling, support groups, education, and financial assistance.

- **Cancer Support Community (cancersupportcommunity.org)**
  Information and support for living with cancer.

- **Cancer.Net (cancer.net)**
  Doctor-approved patient information on the disease, care, emotions, and research from clinical experts.

- **Conquer Cancer (conquer.org)**
  Research, support, and inspirational patient stories of cancer experiences.

- **Cure Magazine (curetoday.com)**
  Cancer updates, research, and education.

- **Get Palliative Care (getpalliativecare.org)**
  Information and provider directory organized by zip code.

- **National Cancer Institute (cancer.gov)**
  Cancer research and information from the
  U.S. government.

- **National Coalition of Cancer Survivorship (canderadvocacy.org)**
  Advocating for quality care for all people touched
  by cancer.

Peer-Support Networks

- **Cancer Hope Network (cancerhopenetwork.org)**
  One-on-one support for adults affected by cancer.

- **I Had Cancer (Ihadcancer.com)**
  An online support community that empowers people to
  take control of life before, during, and after cancer.

- **Imerman Angels (imermanangels.org)**
  Free, personalized, one-on-one support for cancer fighters,
  survivors, and caregivers.

- **Stupid Cancer (stupidcancer.org)**
  The leader in young-adult cancer advocacy, research,
  support, and education.

Organizations Specific to Types of Cancer

- **Colon Cancer Foundation (coloncancerfoundation.org)**
  Information, resources, and support for prevention and care of colon cancer.

- **Idaho2Fly (idaho2fly.org)**
  Support for men with cancer offered through retreats centered on fly fishing.

- **Leukemia and Lymphoma Society (lls.org)**
  Information and resources about blood cancers.

- **Living Beyond Breast Cancer (lbbc.org)**
  Information and support for breast cancer patients.

- **Lungevity (longevity.org)**
  Research, education, and support for lung cancer.

- **Melanoma Research Foundation (melanoma.org)**
  Information, support, and connections to research and care for melanoma and other skin cancers.

- **Share (sharecancersupport.org)**
  Support for women facing breast or ovarian cancer.

- **Us Too (ustoo.org)**
  Information, educational resources, and support services for men with prostate cancer.

- **Women to Women (ocrahope.org)**
  Peer-support program for women with gynecologic cancers.

Other Helpful Resources

- **Well Again (wellagain.org)**
  Inspired coaching through cancer treatment and beyond.

- **A Fresh Chapter (afreshchapter.org)**
  Support for patients, survivors, and caregivers through giving to others.

- **Needy Meds (needymeds.org)**
  Information on programs designed to help those with financial difficulty pay for medications.

ACKNOWLEDGMENTS

As with most things cancer-related, the path between the initial questions asked and this book, which attempts to answer them, was not a straight line. The ideas evolved—with numerous twists and turns and unexpected forks and diversions—as I gained greater understanding along the way. Many people were so generous with their time, their insights, their stories, their contacts, and their encouragement as they helped clear the path and establish the vision realized in these pages. I am grateful to you all.

I particularly would like to thank my contributors, Ann Marie Beddoe, MD, MPH; Sara Pasternak, PhD; and Cristian Zanartu, MD, who, early in our discussions, also recognized the need to provide emotional support to patients and caregivers through the cancer experience. They helped me shape my ideas, contributed so many of their own, and supported my efforts to turn them into a book all while continuing to treat the many patients who count on them every day.

I am so grateful to Shalom Kalnicki, MD and Steve Libutti, MD, whose confidence in me and my research helped to validate my work from the very beginning. Their connections helped expand the scope of the effort, and their constant support and encouragement gave me the conviction to persist over the rocky four years needed to bring it to light.

I am forever indebted to Jonathan Alpert, MD, whose willingness to sit with a total stranger and share insights into the human psychological experience lent further credence to my research. His readiness to make introductions for me opened up a whole new world of understanding. I couldn't have done it without the crash course in neuroscience given to me by his colleagues Kerry Ressler, MD, PhD, and Greg Fricchione, MD; and a similar one in other aspects of the psychological response to cancer shared by Carlos Fernandes-Robles, MD; John Peteet, MD; and Naomi Simon, MD. In the same way, I am indebted to Joe Belanoff, MD and David Spiegel, MD, for the important lessons in cortisol and the stress reaction they so generously provided, and to Alexandra Sansosti, MD for the insights on the immune system and recovery she offered.

I would also like to thank Peter Dottino, MD; Ting Bao, MD; and Martha Eddy, EdD, who patiently conveyed their wisdom and allowed me to present our intact dialogues in the book. And a special thanks to the patients and loving caregivers who were willing to share the most intimate details of their experiences with me and readers everywhere, inviting me into their homes and their lives so that others might suffer a little less.

Thank you to Joanna Barsh and Jennifer Wilcov who guided me through the process of conducting interviews, writing proposals and so many other details of getting published; to Rachelle Sanders, Heidi Diamond, and Gordon Earle who opened up their contact files to make introductions that set off chain reactions of knowledge and connections; and to Judith Nelson, MD, JD, and Molly Lieber, MPH, MSW for their early assistance with my research.

A special thank you to Rachel Justus, Jillian Levinson, and all my fellow Mt. Sinai Woman to Woman peer mentors, as well as to Alyson Moadel, PhD, the Montefiore Einstein BOLD program, and all my fellow BOLD Buddies, for their constant inspiration and support, and for all the important work they do to care for cancer patients in need. Likewise, I am appreciative of the folks at Ovarian Cancer Research Foundation, Global Focus on Cancer, The Max Foundation, and Chai for Cancer for recognizing the importance of my research, making introductions to patients around the world, and for their ongoing support for cancer patients everywhere.

Thank you to my family and friends who volunteered their contacts, introducing me to patients and caregivers who had stories to tell, and a special thanks to those who offered to be early readers and gave me so much encouragement and editorial assistance, including Peter Taback, Fran and Irwin Epstein, Ron Balzan, Eliot Nerenberg, Amy Jaffe, Elizabeth Marek, and Margaret Nordlinger.

Thank you to Kelly Stiles for creating a compelling and informative illustration that captures the essence of *The Big Ordeal* and for adding design sense to the book's digital presence.

Thank you to Jane Taylor for making time amid her own pressing deadlines to proofread my manuscript and correct my endnotes, and to the terrific team at Greenleaf for their enthusiasm and skill in helping me bring the finished product to fruition.

A special thanks to Eric Saltzman, who started it all by sharing his story on a bike at the gym that day, giving me the first inkling of an idea that became this book.

And most importantly, my deepest appreciation to my devoted husband, Charlie, and our fabulous children David and Katharine, whose confidence in me and support for my endeavors are as unending as their love.

NOTES

Introduction

1. Institute of Medicine, *Cancer Care for the Whole Patient: Meeting Psychosocial Health Needs* (Washington, DC: National Academies Press, 2008), doi: 10.17226/11993.

2. R. D. Mehta and A. J. Roth, "Psychiatric Considerations in the Oncology Setting," *CA: A Cancer Journal for Clinicians* 65 (2015): 299–314, doi: 10.3322/caac.21285.

3. A. L. Stanton, J. H. Rowland, and P. A. Ganz, "Life after Diagnosis and Treatment of Cancer in Adulthood: Contributions from Psychosocial Oncology Research," *American Psychologist* 70, no. 2 (2015): 159–74, doi: 10.1037/a0037875.

4. J. Holland, W. Breitbart, P. Jacobson, M. Lederberg, M. Loscalzo, and R. McCorkle, *Psycho-Oncology*, 2nd ed. (Oxford: Oxford University Press, 2010), 3–12.

5. *American Society of Clinical Oncology Educational Book* 38 (May 23, 2018): 813–21, doi: 10.1200/EDBK_201307.

6. A. Grossert, C. Urech, J. Alder, J. Gaab, T. Berger, and V. Hess, "Web-Based Stress Management for Newly Diagnosed Cancer Patients (STREAM-1): A Randomized, Wait-List Controlled Intervention Study," *BMC Cancer* 16 (2016): 838, doi: 10.1186/s12885-016-2866-0.

7. American Cancer Society, *Global Cancer Facts and Figures*, 3rd ed., https://www.cancer.org/content/dam/cancer-org/research/cancer-facts-and-statistics/global-cancer-facts-and-figures/global-cancer-facts-and-figures-3rd-edition.pdf.

8. Brij M. Sood et al., "Patterns of Failure after the Multimodality Treatment of Uterine Papillary Serous Carcinoma," *International Journal of Radiation Oncology • Biology • Physics* 57, no. 1 (2013): 208–16, doi: 10.1016/S0360-3016(03)00531-5.

Chapter 1

1. American Cancer Society, *The History of Cancer: Early History*, https://www.cancer.org/cancer/cancer-basics/history-of-cancer/what-is-cancer.html.

2. National Cancer Institute, *Cancer Statistics: U.S. Cancer Mortality Trends*, https://www.cancer.gov/about-cancer/understanding/statistics.

3. R. L. Siegel, K. D. Miller, and A. Jemal, "Cancer Statistics, 2020," *CA: A Cancer Journal for Clinicians* 70 (2020): 7–30, doi: 10.3322/caac.21590.

4. National Cancer Institute, *Annual Report to the Nation, 2017: Survival*, https://seer.cancer.gov/report_to_nation/

5. G. L. Fricchione, A. Ivkovic, and A. S. Young, *The Science of Stress: Living under Pressure* (Chicago: University of Chicago Press, 2016), 45, https://press.uchicago.edu/ucp/books/book/chicago/S/bo25022182.html.

6. Charissa Andriotti et al., "Cancer, Coping, and Cognition: A Model for the Role of Stress Reactivity in Cancer-Related Cognitive Decline," *Psycho-Oncology* 24, no. 6 (2015): 617–23, doi: 10.1002/pon.3683.

7. F. Gil, G. Costa, I. Hilker, and L. Benito, "First Anxiety, Afterwards Depression: Psychological Distress in Cancer Patients at Diagnosis and after Medical Treatment," *Stress and Health* 28 (2012): 362–67, doi: 10.1002/smi.2445.

8. C. Lai, B. Borrelli, P. Ciurluini, and P. Aceto, "Sharing Information about Cancer with One's Family Is Associated with Improved Quality of Life," *Psycho-Oncology* 26, no. 10 (2017): 1569–75, doi: 10.1002/pon.4334.

9. Thierry Steimer, "The Biology of Fear and Anxiety-Related Behaviors," *Dialogues in Clinical Neuroscience* 4, no. 3 (2002): 231–49.

Chapter 2

1. Betty Chewning et al., "Patient Preferences for Shared Decisions: A Systemic Review," *Patient Education and Counseling* 86, no. 1 (2012): 9–18, doi: 10.1016/j.pec.2011.02.004.

2. C. Radenback et al., "The Interaction of Acute and Chronic Stress Impairs Model-Based Behavioral Control," *Psychoneuroendocrinology* (December 2, 2014): 268–80.

3. B. De Martino, D. Kumaran, B. Seymour, and R. J. Dolan, "Frames, Biases, and Rational Decision-Making in the Human Brain," *Science* 313, no. 5787 (August 2006): 684–87, doi: 10.1126/science.1128356.

4. E. A. Phelps, K. M. Lempert, and P. Sokol-Hessner, "Emotion and Decision-Making: Multiple Modulatory Neural Circuits," *Annual Review of Neuroscience* 37 (2014): 263–87, doi: 10.1146/annurev-neuro-071013-014119.

5. S. Nagappan, "The Deciding Brain and the Effects of Stress," *Harvard Neuro Blog* (June 21, 2016), https://harvardneuro.wordpress.com/2016/06/21/the-deciding-brain-and-the-effects-of-stress/.

6. G. S. Shields, J. C. Lam, B. C. Trainor, and A. P. Yonelinas, "Exposure to Acute Stress Enhances Decision-Making Competence: Evidence for the Role of DHEA," Psychoneuroendocrinology, 2016 May; 67:51-60. doi: 10.1016/j.psyneuen.2016.01.031.

7. P. Morgado, N. Sousa, and J. J. Cerqueira, "The Impact of Stress in Decision-Making in the Context of Uncertainty," *Journal of Neuroscience Research* 93 (2015): 839–47, doi: 10.1002/jnr.23521.

8. C. A. Bryce and S. B. Floresco, "Perturbations in Effort-Related Decision Making Driven by Acute Stress and Corticotropin Releasing Factor," *Neuropsychopharmacology* 41 (2016): 2147–59, doi: 10.1038/npp.2016.15.

9. M. E. Authement et al., "A Role for Corticotropin-Releasing Factor Signaling in the Lateral Habenula and Its Modulation by Early-Life Stress," *Science Signaling* (March 6, 2018): 520, doi: 10.1126/scisignal.aan6480.

Chapter 3

1. *Cancer Research Institute Immunotherapy Timeline,* http://cancerresearch.org/immunotherapy/timeline-of-progress.

2. American Cancer Society, *History of Cancer*, https://www.cancer.org /cancer/cancer-basics/history-of-cancer.html.

3. American Cancer Society, *Global Cancer Facts and Figures*, https://www. cancer.org/research/cancer-facts-statistics.html.

4. J. M. Greenblatt, "The Brain on Fire: Inflammation and Depression," *Psychology Today* (November 23, 2011), https://www.psychologytoday.com /us/blog/the-breakthrough-depression-solution/201111/the-brain-fire -inflammation-and-depression.

5. A. H. Miller and C. L. Raison, "The Role of Inflammation in Depression: From Evolutionary Imperative to Modern Treatment Target," *National Review of Immunology* 16, no. 1 (2016): 22–34, doi:10.1038/nri.2015.5

6. N. C. Donner et al., "Two Models of Inescapable Stress Increase *tph2* mRNA Expression in the Anxiety-Related Dorsomedial Part of the Dorsal Raphe Nucleus," *Neurobiology of Stress* (January 2018): 68–81, doi: 10.1016/j.ynstr.2018.01.003.

7. R. S. Thompson et al., "Effects of Stressor Controllability on Diurnal Physiological Rhythms," *Physiological Behavior* (March 15, 2013): 32–39, doi: 10.1016/j.physbeh.2013.02.009.

8. T. A. Ahles, J. C. Root, and E. L. Ryan, "Cancer- and Cancer Treatment– Associated Cognitive Change: An Update on the State of the Science," *Journal of Clinical Oncology* 30, no. 30 (October 20, 2012): 3675–86, doi: 10.1200/JCO.2012.43.0116.

9. X. M. Wang et al., "Chemobrain: A Critical Review and Causal Hypothesis of Link between Cytokines and Epigenetic Reprogramming Associated with Chemotherapy," *Cytokine* 72, no. 1 (March 2015): 86–96, doi: 10.1016/j.cyto.2014.12.006.

Chapter 4

1. Mehta and Roth, "Psychiatric Considerations."

2. Stanton, Rowland, and Ganz, "Life after Diagnosis."

3. J. Carter et al., "Interventions to Address Sexual Problems in People with Cancer: American Society of Clinical Oncology Clinical Practice Guideline Adaptation of Cancer Care Ontario Guideline," *Journal of Clinical Oncology* 36, no. 5 (February 10, 2018): 492–511, doi: 10.1200/

JCO.2017.75.8995; D. S. Dizon, S. Suzin, and S. McIlvenna, "Sexual Health as a Survivorship Issue for Female Cancer Survivors," *Oncologist* 12 (2014): 202–10, doi: 10.1634/theoncologist.2013-0302.

4. M. R. Krause et al., "Sexual Dysfunction in Males with Chronic Hepatitis C and Antiviral Therapy: Interferon-Induced Functional Androgen Deficiency or Depression?" *Journal of Endocrinology* 185, no. 2 (2005): 345–52, doi: 10.1677/joe.1.06007.

5. J. Veldhuis et al., "Proinflammatory Cytokine Infusion Attenuates LH's Feedforward on Testosterone Secretion: Modulation by Age," *Journal of Clinical Endocrinology and Metabolism* 101, vol. 2 (2016): 539–49, https://academic.oup.com/jcem/article/101/2/539/2810786.

6. E. Bini et al., "The Implication of Pro-Inflammatory Cytokines in the Impaired Production of Gonadal Androgens by Patients with Pulmonary Tuberculosis," *Tuberculosis* 95, no. 6 (December 2015): 701–706, doi: 10.1016/j.tube.2015.06.002.

7. J. A. Albaugh et al., "Sexual Dysfunction and Intimacy for Ostomates," *Clinical Rectal Surgery* 30 (2017): 201–206, doi: 10.1055/s-0037-1598161.

8. S. C. Notari et al., "Women's Experiences of Sexual Function in the Early Weeks of Breast Cancer Treatment," *European Journal of Cancer Care* (2018): 27:e12607, doi: 10.1111/ecc.12607.

9. K. G. Bennett, J. Qi, H. M. Kim, J. B. Hamill, A. L. Pusic, and E. G. Wilkins, "Comparison of 2-Year Complication Rates among Common Techniques for Postmastectomy Breast Reconstruction," *JAMA Surgery* (June 20, 2018): 901–8, https://jamanetwork.com/journals/jamasurgery/fullarticle/2685264.

10. K. A. Donovan et al., "Effect of Androgen Deprivation Therapy on Sexual Function and Bother in Men with Prostate Cancer: A Controlled Comparison," *Psycho-Oncology* 27 (2018): 316–24, doi: 10.1002/pon.4463.

11. W. Surbeck, G. Herbet, and H. Dufau, "Sexuality after Surgery for Diffuse Low-Grade Glioma," *Neuro-Oncology* 17, no. 4 (2015): 574–79, doi: 10.1093/neuonc/nou326.

12. L. R. Schover et al., "Sexual Dysfunction and Infertility as Late Effects of Cancer Treatment," *European Journal of Cancer,* EJC Supplements 12 (2014): 41–53, doi: 10.1016/j.ejcsup.2014.03.004.

13. L. M. Walker, P. Santos-Inglesias, and J. Robinson, "Mood, Sexuality, and Relational Intimacy after Starting Androgen Deprivation Therapy: Implications for Couples," *Supportive Care in Cancer* (May 2018): 3835–42,

https://doi.org/10.1007/s00520-018-4251-9; Dizon, Suzin, and McIlvenna, "Sexual Health."

14. A. Villa et al., "Estrogen Accelerates the Resolution of Inflammation in Macrophagic Cells," *Nature Scientific Reports* 5 (2015): 15224, doi: 10.1038/ srep15224.

15. Dizon, Suzin, and McIlvenna, "Sexual Health."

Chapter 5

1. L. Koch, L. Jansen, H. Brenner, and V. Arndt, "Fear of Recurrence and Disease Progression in Long Term Cancer Survivors—A Systemic Review of Quantitative Studies," *Psycho-Oncology* 22 (2013): 1–11, doi: 10.1002/ pon.3022.

2. C. A. Thompson et al., "Surveillance CT Scans Are a Source of Anxiety and Fear of Recurrence in Long-Term Lymphoma Survivors," *Annals of Oncology* 21 (2010): 2262–66, doi: 10.1093/annonc/mdq215.

3. J. M. Bauml et al., "Scan-Associated Distress in Lung Cancer: Quantifying the Impact of 'Scanxiety,'" *Lung Cancer* 100 (2016 October): 110–13, doi: 10.1016/j.lungcan.2016.08.002; K. M. Gil et al., "Triggers of Uncertainty about Recurrence and Long-Term Treatment Side Effects in Older African American and Caucasian Breast Cancer Survivors," Oncol Nurs Forum, 2004; 31(3): 633–639. doi:10.1188/04.onf.633–639

4. A. Grilo et al., "Anxiety in Cancer Patients during ^{18}F-FDG PET/CT Low Dose: A Comparison of Anxiety Levels Before and After Imaging Studies," *Nursing Research and Practice* (March 14, 2017): 3057495, doi: 10.1155/2017/3057495.

5. M. J. Cordova, M. B. Riba, and D. Spiegel, "Post-Traumatic Stress Disorder and Cancer," *Lancet Psychiatry* 4, no. 4 (2017): 330–38, doi: 10.1016/S2215-0366(17)30014-7.

6. Ibid.

7. T. T. Levin and Y. Alici, "Anxiety Disorders," in *Psycho-Oncology,* edited by Jimmie C. Holland et al., Oxford University Press, 2nd ed., 2010, pg. 324.

8. F. Gil et al., "First Anxiety, Afterwards Depression."

9. H. J. Tan et al., "The Relationship between Intolerance of Uncertainty and Anxiety in Men on Active Surveillance for Prostate Cancer," *Journal of Urology* 196, no. 6 (2016): 1724–30, doi: 10.1016/j.juro.2016.01.108.

10. L. Castelli et al., "The Neurobiological Basis of the Distress Thermometer: A PET Study in Cancer Patients," *Stress & Health* 31, no. 3 (August 2015): 197–201, doi: 10.1002/smi.2546.

11. Cordova, Riba, and Spiegel, "Post-Traumatic Stress Disorder."

12. C. Miaskowski et al., "Cytokine Gene Variations Associated with Trait and State Anxiety in Oncology Patients and Their Family Caregivers," *Supportive Care in Cancer* 23, no. 4 (2015): 953–65, doi: 10.1007/s00520-014-2443-5.

13. Ibid.

14. Cordova, Riba, and Spiegel, "Post-Traumatic Stress Disorder."; D. L. Hall et al., "Mind-Body Interventions for Fear of Cancer Recurrence: A Systemic Review and Meta-Analysis," *Psycho-Oncology* (2018): 1–13, doi: 10.1002/pon.4757.

15. M. K. Bhasin et al., "Relaxation Response Induces Temporal Transcriptome Changes in Energy Metabolism, Insulin Secretion, and Inflammatory Pathways," *PLoS ONE* 8, no. 5 (2013): e62817, doi: 10.1371 /journal.pone.0062817.

Chapter 6

1. M. Colleoni, Z. Sun, K. N. Price et al., "Annual Hazard Rates of Recurrence for Breast Cancer during 24 Years of Follow-Up: Results from the International Breast Cancer Study Group Trials I to V," *Journal of Clinical Oncology* 34, no. 9 (2016): 927–35, doi: 10.1200/JCO.2015.62.3504.

2. N. Donin et al., "Risk of Second Primary Malignancies among Cancer Survivors in the United States, 1992 through 2008," *Cancer* 122 (2016): 3075–86, doi: 10.1002/cncr.30164.

3. O. W. Foley, J. A. Rauh-Hain, and M. G. del Carmen, "Recurrent Epithelial Ovarian Cancer: An Update on Treatment," *Oncology* (Williston Park) 27, no. 4 (2013): 288–98, https://www.cancernetwork.com/view /recurrent-epithelial-ovarian-cancer-update-treatment.

4. B. M. Scarborough and C. B. Smith, "Optimal Pain Management for Patients with Cancer in the Modern Era," *CA: A Cancer Journal for Clinicians* 68, no. 3 (2018): 182–96, doi: 10.3322/caac.21453; J. A. Paice, "Navigating Cancer Pain Management in the Midst of the Opioid

Epidemic," *Oncology* (Williston Park) 32, no. 8 (2018): 386–403, https://www.cancernetwork.com/view/navigating-cancer-pain-management-midst-opioid-epidemic.

5. W. Leppert et al., "Pathophysiology and Clinical Characteristics of Pain in Most Common Locations in Cancer Patients," *Journal of Physiology and Pharmacology* 67, no. 6 (2016): 787–99.

6. O. Paulsen, B. Laird, N. Aass et al., "The Relationship between Pro-inflammatory Cytokines and Pain, Appetite, and Fatigue in Patients with Advanced Cancer," *PLoS ONE* 12, no. 5 (2017): e0177620, doi: 10.1371/journal.pone.0177620.

7. T. G. Smith, A. N. Troeschel, K. M. Castro et al., "Perceptions of Patients with Breast and Colon Cancer of the Management of Cancer-Related Pain, Fatigue, and Emotional Distress in Community Oncology," *Journal of Clinical Oncology* 37, no. 19 (2019): 1666–76, doi: 10.1200/JCO.18.01579.

Chapter 7

1. Surveillance, Epidemiology, and End Results (SEER) Program, "SEER*Stat Database: Mortality-All COD, Total US (1990–2017)," National Cancer Institute, Division of Cancer Control and Population Sciences, Surveillance Research Program (2019), https://seer.cancer.gov/csr/1975_2017/.

2. Siegel, Miller, and Jemal, "Cancer Statistics, 2020."

3. J. R. Lunney, J. Lyon et al., "Patterns of Functional Decline at the End of Life," *JAMA* 289, no. 18 (2003): 39–44, doi: 10.1001/jama.289.18.2387.

4. H. Seow, L. Barbera, R. Sutradhar et al., "Trajectory of Performance Status and Symptom Scores for Patients with Cancer during the Last Six Months of Life," *Journal of Clinical Oncology* 29, no. 9 (2011): 1151–58, doi: 10.1200/JCO.2010.30.7173.; D. Hui, R. dos Santos, G. B. Chisholm, and E. Bruera, "Symptom Expression in the Last Seven Days of Life among Cancer Patients Admitted to Acute Palliative Care Units," *Journal of Pain and Symptom Management* 50, no. 4 (October 2015): 488–94, doi: 10.1016/j.jpainsymman.2014.09.003.

5. K. Fearon et al., "Cancer Cachexia: Mediators, Signaling, and Metabolic Pathways," *Cell Metabolism* 16, no. 2 (2012): 153–66, doi: 10.1016/j.cmet.2012.06.011.

6. D. Hui et al., "Clinical Signs of Impending Death in Cancer Patients," *Oncologist* 19, no. 6 (2014): 681–87, doi: 10.1634/theoncologist.2013-0457.

7. Ibid.

8. S. Pautex, P. Vayne-Bossert, S. Jamme et al., "Anatomopathological Causes of Death in Patients with Advanced Cancer: Association with the Use of Anticoagulation and Antibiotics at the End of Life," *Journal of Palliative Medicine* 16, no. 6 (2013): 669–74, doi: 10.1089/jpm.2012.0369.

9. Sebastian Bruera et al., "Variations in Vital Signs in the Last Days of Life in Patients with Advanced Cancer," *Journal of Pain and Symptom Management* 48, no. 4 (2014): 510–17, doi: 10.1016/j.jpainsymman.2013.10.019.

10. Seow, Barbera, and Sutradhar, "Trajectory of Performance Status."

11. Bruera et al., "Variations in Vital Signs."

12. J. H. Lotterman, G. A. Bonanno, and I. Galatzer-Levy, "The Heterogeneity of Long-Term Grief Reactions," *Journal of Affective Disorders* 167, no. 1 (October 2014): 12–19, doi: 10.1016/j.jad.2014.05.048.

13. E. An, C. Lo, S. Hales, C. Zimmermann, and G. Rodin, "Demoralization and Death Anxiety in Advanced Cancer," *Psycho-Oncology* 27, no. 11 (2018): 2566–72, doi: 10.1002/pon.4843.

14. S. Vehling and D. W. Kissane, "Existential Distress in Cancer: Alleviating Suffering from Fundamental Loss and Change," *Psycho-Oncology* 27, no. 11 (2018): 2525–30, doi: 10.1002/pon.4872.

Chapter 8

1. M. Fitch, S. Zomer, G. Lockwood et al., "Experiences of Adult Cancer Survivors in Transitions," *Supportive Care in Cancer* 27, no. 8 (2019): 2977–86, doi: 10.1007/s00520-018-4605-3.

2. M. D. Stubblefield, K. H. Schmitz, and K. K. Ness, "Physical Functioning and Rehabilitation for the Cancer Survivor," *Seminars in Oncology* 40, no. 6 (2013): 784–95, doi: 10.1053/j.seminoncol.2013.09.008.

3. J. M. Reinke and H. Sorg, "Wound Repair and Regeneration," *European Surgical Review* 49 (2012): 35–43, doi: 10.1159/000339613.

4. W. G. Payne, D. K. Naidu, C. K. Wheeler, D. Barkoe, M. Mentis, R. E. Salas, D. J. Smith Jr., and M. C. Robson, "Wound Healing in Patients with Cancer," *Eplasty* 8 (January 11, 2008): e9.

5. S. He and N. E. Sharpless, "Senescence in Health and Disease," *Cell* 169 (2017): 1000–11, doi: 10.1016/j.cell.2017.05.015.

6. M. Gawaz and S. Vogel, "Platelets in Tissue Repair: Control of Apoptosis and Interactions with Regenerative Cells," *Blood* 122, no. 15 (2013): 2550–54, doi: 10.1182/blood-2013-05-468694.

7. F. Brenet, P. Kermani, R. Spektor, S. Rafii, and J. M. Scandura, "TGF*b* Restores Hematopoietic Homeostasis after Myelosuppressive Chemotherapy," *Journal of Experimental Medicine* 210, no. 3 (2013): 623–39, doi: 10.1084/jem.20121610.

8. V. Syed, "TGF-b Signaling in Cancer," *Journal of Cellular Biochemistry* 117 (2016): 1279–87, doi: 10.1002/jcb.25496.

9. G. R. Morrow, P. L. R. Andrews, J. T. Hickok, J. A. Roscoe, and S. Matteson, "Fatigue Associated with Cancer and Its Treatment," *Supportive Care in Cancer* 10 (2002): 389–98, doi: 10.1007/s005200100293.

10. F. W. Booth, C. K. Roberts, J. P. Thyfault, G. N. Ruegsegger, and R. G. Toedebusch, "Role of Inactivity in Chronic Diseases: Evolutionary Insight and Pathophysiological Mechanisms," *Physiology Review* 97 (2017): 1351–1402, doi: 10.1152/physrev.00019.2016.

11. Morrow et al., "Fatigue Associated with Cancer."

12. Payne et al., "Wound Healing."

13. L. N. Saligan, K. Olson, K. Filler, D. Larkin, F. Cramp, S. Yennurajalingam, C. P. Escalante et al., "The Biology of Cancer-Related Fatigue: A Review of the Literature," *Supportive Care in Cancer* 23, no. 8 (2015): 2461–78, doi: 10.1007/s00520-015-2763-0.

14. Booth et al., "Role of Inactivity."

15. R. J. Thomas, S. A. Kenfield, and A. Jimenez, "Exercise-Induced Biochemical Changes and Their Potential Influence on Cancer: A Scientific Review," *British Journal of Sports Medicine* 51, no. 8 (2017): 640–44, doi: 10.1136/bjsports-2016-096343.

16. National Cancer Institute, *Physical Activity and Cancer Fact Sheet*, https://www.cancer.gov/about-cancer/causes-prevention/risk/obesity/physical-activity-fact-sheet.

Chapter 9

1. Stanton, Rowland, and Ganz, "Life after Diagnosis."

2. Ibid.

3. Ibid.

4. S. J. Russo, J. W. Murrough, M. H. Han, D. S. Charney, and E. J. Nestler, "Neurobiology of Resilience," *Nature Neuroscience* 15, no. 11 (2012): 1475–84, doi: 10.1038/nn.3234.

5. F. Cathomas, J. W. Murrough, E. J. Nestler, M. H. Han, and S. J. Russo, "Neurobiology of Resilience: Interface between Mind and Body," *Biological Psychiatry* 86 (2019): 410–20, doi: 10.1016/j.biopsych.2019.04.011.

6. Russo et al., "Neurobiology of Resilience."

7. B. Patoine, "The Resilient Brain," *Dana Foundation*, https://www.dana.org/article/the-neurobiology-of-resilience/.

8. Russo et al., "Neurobiology of Resilience."; D. E. J. Linden, "How Psychotherapy Changes the Brain: The Contribution of Functional Neuroimaging," *Molecular Psychiatry* 11 (2006): 528–38, doi: 10.1038/sj.mp.4001816.

ABOUT THE AUTHOR

Cynthia Hayes has been preparing her whole life to write *The Big Ordeal*. She learned the basics of interviewing, synthesizing information, finding the headlines, and telling a story as a journalist early in her career. After a brief interruption to earn an MBA from Harvard Business School, Cynthia spent twenty-five years as a management consultant. In that role, success depended on her ability to jump into new topics, ask sensitive questions, understand specialized information, and turn complex findings into a compelling narrative.

Shortly prior to her own diagnosis, Cynthia resigned from Montefiore Medical Center in New York, where for three years she had served as vice president and chief marketing officer, focused on telling stories of health and recovery. While at Montefiore, she gained a deeper understanding of medicine and had the opportunity to build relationships with cancer professionals and other experts who helped her write *The Big Ordeal*.

When Cynthia is not on the tennis court or writing, she mentors patients going through gynecologic cancer as part of a program called Woman to Woman at Mount Sinai Hospital in New York, and serves as a BOLD Buddy peer mentor to patients receiving care at the Montefiore Einstein Center for Cancer Care in the Bronx. Cynthia also serves on the board of Moving For Life, a dance exercise program to support cancer recovery, and Global Focus on Cancer, which provides education and support for patients in developing countries.

The author lives in New York City with her fabulous husband, Charlie Cummings, two amazing adult children, David and Katharine, and their adoring shih tzu, Horatio, who has sat at her feet through multiple drafts and countless rounds of edits.

Made in the USA
Middletown, DE
19 November 2021

52912667R00158